Manual of Cardiorespiratory Critical Care

Manual of Cardiorespiratory Critical Care

F. Guzman M., MD, IGACS
A. Hedley Brown, MB, MS, FRCS
M. Been, MB, FRCP
S. Cook, MB, BS, MRCP(UK), FFARCS
C. Wren, MB, ChB, MRCP
D. Richens, MB, FRCS
Freeman Hospital,
Newcastle upon Tyne.

Royal Victoria Infirmary,
Newcastle upon Tyne

Butterworths
London   Boston   Singapore   Sydney   Toronto   Wellington

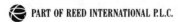 PART OF REED INTERNATIONAL P.L.C.

First published 1989

© Butterworth & Co. (Publishers) Ltd, 1989

British Library Cataloguing in Publication Data

Manual of cardiorespiratory critical care.
  1. Man. Heart. Diseases. Intensive care
  I. Guzman, F.
  616.1'2028

  ISBN 0-407-01253-2

Library of Congress Cataloging-in-Publication Data

Manual of cariorespiratory critical care/F. Guzman M. . . . [et al].
    p.   cm.
  Bibliography: p.
  Includes index.
    1. Cardiopulmonary system–Diseases–Treatment–Handbooks, manuals, etc.   2. Critical care medicine–Handbooks, manuals, etc.   3. Cardiopulmonary system–Surgery–Handbooks, manual, etc.
  I. Guzman M., Fernando.
  [DNLM: 1. Critical Care–handbooks.   2. Heart Diseases–therapy–handbooks.   3. Respiratory Tract Diseases–therapy–handbooks. WG 39 M294]
  RC702.M36   1989
  616.1'2028–dc20

Photoset by Butterworths Litho Preparation Department
Printed and bound in England by Page Bros. Ltd, Norwich, Norfolk

Main editors

A. Hedley Brown, MB, MS, FRCS
Consultant Cardiothoracic Surgeon,
Freeman Hospital,
Newcastle upon Tyne

Fernando Guzman M., MD, IGACS
Senior Registrar in Cardiothoracic Surgery,
Freeman Hospital,
Newcastle upon Tyne; Consultant Cardiothoracic Surgeon,
Centro Medico de Los Andes,
Fundacion Santa Fe de Bogota,
Bogota,
Colombia,
South America

Steven Cook, MB, BS, MRCP (UK), FFARCS
Consultant in Anaesthesia and Intensive Care,
Royal Victoria Infirmary,
Newcastle upon Tyne

Christopher Wren, MB, ChB, MRCP
Senior Registrar in Paediatric Cardiology,
Freeman Hospital,
Newcastle upon Tyne

David Richens, MB, FRCS
Registrar in Cardiothoracic Surgery,
Freeman Hospital,
Newcastle upon Tyne

V

Contributors

Medical staff

R. Bray
I. Conacher
D. Dougenis
C. J. Hilton
A. Kirk
D. McLeod
G. N. Morritt
S. Naik
D. Veale
C. Vallis

Nursing and technical staff

J. Boyack
B. Cooper
S. Farr
B. Hallam
I. Knox
L. Llewellyn
B. M. McNally SRN
E. Middleton
M. Pitt
A. Townsend
C. Walton
A. Wilson

Preface

This book is directed at those who are at the 'sharp end' of the very acute medicine and surgery practised nowadays. Its emphasis is on practical instant help in acute situations and it is intended more as a source of reference than to be read through. The subsections are therefore very short and self-contained for quick perusal under fraught circumstances and for this reason there may be some duplication, especially as there are some overviews followed by details of the procedures recommended in separate small chapters, e.g. the management of balloon counterpulsation.

We have tried to provide plenty of usable numbers and to give details, but hope that the general overviews balance somewhat the methodological approach to the advice given elsewhere, where one might be in some fear of 'doctoring by numbers'.

With all of the technical advice it is difficult to deliver perfect prose but we have tried to avoid too many solecisms and hope that this will make the burden of reading a little lighter; we hope withal to be easing the burden of the actual work that has to be done. This is therefore a book for the workplace and we hope it will find its home in many such frontlines of technical medicine and surgery.

Contents

Cardiac medicine

Physiological basis of cardiac critical care

Myocardial blood supply

The right and left coronary arteries originate from the right and left sinuses of Valsalva situated just above the aortic valve. From the left sinus of Valsalva arises the left main stem which, after a variable interval, divides into the (left) anterior descending (LAD) and circumflex (Cx) arteries. These arteries run along the epicardial surface of the heart and give off branches which penetrate and supply the myocardium.

The left anterior descending artery is prognostically very important because it supplies most of the left ventricular myocardium. It gives rise to (often large) diagonal branches and to septal branches. The diagonal branches also lie on the epicardial surface but the septal vessels travel into the interventricular muscle (and so are less amenable to bypass grafting). The circumflex artery supplies the lateral wall of the left ventricle, including papillary muscle. It may give rise to the posterior descending artery and is then called 'dominant'.

The right coronary artery supplies the right ventricle and a variable amount of the inferior left ventricular myocardium. It is usually the dominant artery (giving rise to the posterior descending artery and a posterior left ventricular branch).

Variations in this pattern of coronary arterial supply may be due to:

1. Variable dominance of right and circumflex coronary arteries.
2. Presence of intermediate artery (between LAD and Cx).
3. Collateral circulation from other coronary arteries.
4. Left ventricular branch.
5. Aberrant origin of a coronary artery.

After efficient oxygen extraction by the myocardium, the venous return enters the right side of the heart via the coronary sinus and anterior cardiac veins.

Conducting system blood supply

The blood supply to the sinus node is predominantly from the right coronary artery. The atrioventricular (AV) nodal supply is usually from the right coronary artery but this may be supplied by the circumflex. (This explains why inferior infarcts are frequently associated with bradycardias.) The bundle of His runs in the interventricular septum which is supplied by the left anterior descending artery.

Coronary blood flow

At rest, coronary blood flow is normally around 175 ml/min, divided unequally between the three arteries, and flow may be maintained even where stenotic lesions are severe. During exercise, coronary flow increases greatly and stenotic lesions, particularly those greater than 70%, severely restrict the necessary increase in flow.

Factors which may affect coronary flow are:

1. Severity of stenosis.
2. Coronary arterial tone/spasm.
3. Aortic pressure (particularly diastolic).
4. Heart rate and duration of diastole.
5. Intramyocardial pressure.
6. Viscosity.
7. Myocardial bridging (constriction of a coronary artery during myocardial contraction): some flow does occur during systole but bridging usually only results in ischaemia when it is so severe as completely to occlude the vessel with each contraction.

Viewing coronary angiograms

At least two projections of each vessel are usually taken to allow more accurate interpretation as lesions may, on the one hand, be missed using a single projection and, on the other hand, overestimate the severity of stenosis in a particular view.

Distinguishing between the LAD and Cx arteries at angiography requires knowledge of the projections used and some experience. Left-sided views (left anterior oblique and left lateral) show the LAD on the left side of the projection. Slightly more difficult is the differentiation between diagonal and septal branches of the LAD. Here, the most helpful view is usually the left anterior oblique projection with cranial tilt. The LAD travels down in a slightly leftward direction, with septal vessels coming off to the left and diagonal vessels to the right. The circumflex is shown to be clearly separate by travelling rightwards before curving down towards the apex.

Cardiac function

The normal cardiac output at rest is about 5 litres per minute. Cardiac output is related to heart rate and stroke volume.

$$CO = HR \times SV$$

Stroke volume is primarily determined by three factors:

1. Preload.
2. Afterload.
3. Contractility.

Preload is the term used to reflect ventricular filling and is usually expressed as the pressure at end of diastole. This and ventricular compliance dictate the volume of blood in the ventricle just before ventricular contraction, i.e. ventricular loading.

Direct or indirect measurement of the left ventricular end-diastolic pressure (LVEDP) is often of great help in hypotensive patients. A low LVEDP indicates that fluid should be administered (providing there is no mitral stenosis) to allow adequate filling of the left ventricle. If the LVEDP is high, then a combination of diuretic and inotropic support will usually be required.

Inadequate preload may also be the result of loss of either atrial contraction or of AV synchrony. In both cases, the atrial contribution to ventricular filling (up to 25% of cardiac output) is lost. Inadequate filling may also occur with rapid tachycardia where there is insufficient time for ventricular relaxation before the next systole.

Afterload is the resistance the heart pumps against in order to eject blood. This is a combination of aortic impedance and peripheral arteriolar resistance.

A rise in peripheral vascular resistance reduces ejection fraction and results in a rise in the wall stress of the ventricle, increasing the oxygen requirement for ejection.

The conducting system

The electrical system of the heart provides optimal timing and rate of contraction of cardiac chambers. The specialised cells which make up the conducting system differ from other muscle cells because they depolarise spontaneously. Normally the sinus node has the fastest rate of depolarisation and is therefore the cardiac 'pacemaker'; it is situated in the right atrium close to the junction with the superior vena cava.

Discharge of the sinus node leads to depolarisation spreading through the atria and this atrial activity is seen in the ECG as the P wave. (Physiologically, this maximises end-diastolic ventricular filling or preload.)

The wave of electrical activity then reaches the AV node – situated just above the tricuspid valve – and then travels along specialised pathways. On leaving the AV node, the impulse passes rapidly along the bundle of His, situated in the interventricular septum, before dividing into the right and left bundle branches. This activity does not register on the standard ECG but occurs during the isoelectric phase between the end of the P wave and the start of the QRS complex. (Direct intracardiac measurement of the electrical activity can record a spike from the His bundle.)

Once the ventricular muscle itself begins to depolarise, spreading from the endocardium to epicardium, electrical activity is detected as the QRS complex.

Cardiac investigations in ITU

Electrocardiograph (ECG) monitor (single lead)

The ECG monitor in ITU usually provides a real-time image of a single electrocardiographic lead. Some monitors have a second line which allows storage of one screen length of ECG tracing. Ideally, monitors should be able to give a printout of the tracing. This allows more accurate interpretation of arrhythmias and provides documentation of events which may otherwise become clouded with time.

The purpose of ECG monitoring is to provide rapid detection of significant changes in cardiac rhythm. Serious arrhythmias will usually trigger the monitor's alarm by detecting either a rise or fall in ventricular rate or amplitude outside preset limits. It has the additional advantage of giving an instant read-out of heart rate so that unexpected changes in heart rate, such as sinus tachycardia, are easily appreciated.

It is important to realise that the single lead system is very insensitive at detecting ST-T wave changes, such as those occurring during myocardial ischaemia. Furthermore, the monitor may falsely suggest changes which are simply due to alteration in a patient's position or respiratory motion. For this reason, it is important that daily 12-lead ECGs are performed and that these are repeated with any significant change in the patient's clinical condition. Chest pain following cardiac surgery is often difficult to evaluate but ischaemia and infarction may be clearly shown by appropriate use of electrocardiography.

Central venous pressure (or jugular venous pulse; JVP)

Much of the information available from a central venous line can be obtained by careful inspection of the JVP. However, patients in ITU are usually lying flat and it is impractical to alter their position every time the measurement is required. Central venous catheters can be passed from any accessible vein to the right atrium.

The commonly used routes along with their advantages and disadvantages, are shown in Table 1.1.

Table 1.1 Routes for insertion of central venous catheters

Vein	Safety and comments
Jugular	Percutaneous approach; safe
Subclavian	Percutaneous approach; quick
	Supraclavicular or infraclavicular but risk of: pneumothorax subclavian artery puncture air embolism
Antecubital	Percutaneous approach or cut-down; safe
Femoral	When other veins inaccessible; unusual

The venous pressure can be measured by assessing the height (in centimetres) a column of saline (or water) reaches above the level of the mid-right atrium or by a pressure transducer which gives a value in millimetres of mercury.

$$1\,cmH_2O = 1/1.36\,mmHg \text{ or } 1\,mmHg = 1.36\,cmH_2O$$

Although measurement of the CVP may be of help in fluid balance control, readings must not be viewed in isolation. While a negative CVP will indicate hypovolaemia, elevation of the venous pulse has a number of different causes which can be determined with additional information.

Causes of elevated CVP

1. Right heart failure, e.g. right ventricular dysfunction, tricuspid valve disease or secondary to pulmonary hypertension, pulmonary emboli or left heart failure.
2. Myocardial restriction.
3. Pericardial effusion or constriction.

It is important to note that the CVP may be normal even when left heart failure is severe and so is not a substitute for wedge pressure measurements when these are indicated. Similarly, with right ventricular infarction the CVP may be elevated but left atrial pressure may be low and the left ventricle underfilled. The waveform of the CVP may provide helpful information.

Arterial pressure trace (or blood pressure)

Continuous display of an arterial pressure wave is of considerable assistance in the postoperative management of cardiothoracic patients. It provides early warnings of problems, allows rapid adjustment of vasoactive drugs to assist in optimisation of haemodynamics, and blood pressure measurements are more accurate.

In many cases these advantages outweigh the risks of introducing an intra-arterial catheter. Most commonly the radial artery is used, with the cannula connected to a transducer via a fluid-filled tube. As with all intravascular catheters, it is essential that the cannula and attached tubing is free of blood or air to prevent embolism or thrombosis and damping of the tracing.

Pulmonary artery wedge pressure

Monitoring of right heart pressures and wedge pressure is performed using a Swan–Ganz catheter. The route of insertion is similar to that used for CVP measurements but the catheter is advanced further into the right ventricle, main pulmonary artery and right or left pulmonary artery. A balloon situated close to the tip of the catheter assists in its passage as it tends to be carried in the correct path by blood flowing through the right heart. Once in place the balloon should be deflated. The correct position is obtained when a pulmonary artery tracing is seen with the balloon deflated and a 'wedge' tracing (left atrial pattern) with the balloon inflated.

In the absence of pulmonary disease, both the PA diastolic and wedge pressure reflect the pressure in the left atrium. In the absence of obstruction at the mitral valve these pressures at the end of diastole reflect the left ventricular end-diastolic pressure ('filling pressure', see p. 3).

Measurement of the filling pressure provides the most accurate assessment of the requirement for fluid or therapy such as vasodilators. This is particularly useful in patients who are hypotensive. If the LVEDP is low then fluid is required, whereas if the LVEDP is high then vasodilators, diuretics or inotropes are required (irrespective of right atrial pressures).

Cardiac output

Measurement of the cardiac output can be of help in diagnosis and is particularly important when considering other haemodynamic indices such as valvular gradients. In order to calculate valve orifice area it is necessary to know the cardiac output. In ITU, the cardiac output is usually measured by means of a thermodilution (Swan–Ganz) catheter. This works by measuring the curve of the temperature change caused by injecting fluid of a known volume and temperature. The (often cooled) dextrose or saline is injected into the right atrial port and the temperature change detected by the thermistor at the catheter tip. The lower the cardiac output, the longer it will take for the fluid (which is cooler than the circulating blood) to drop the temperature at the thermistor and for it subsequently to rise again. The rate of injection of fluid is clearly important and, to reduce variability, a power injection gun is often used.

Owing to frequent variability in measurements it is important to ensure that three consecutive readings give values within 10% of each other.

Cross-sectional echocardiography (+ Doppler)

In a postoperative patient where there is haemodynamic deterioration then echocardiography can be of value in determining the cause. It is very sensitive at detecting pericardial fluid and so may help confirm tamponade. Additionally, echocardiography provides information about myocardial contraction. For example, in a patient who becomes hypotensive following coronary artery bypass graft (CABG), poor ventricular function may suggest early graft closure, while if ventricular function remained good, alternative diagnoses such as blood loss or pulmonary embolism would have to be considered.

In patients undergoing valvular surgery, Doppler examination can confirm normal prosthetic function or identify regurgitation or obstruction. Occasionally, patients with previous valvular surgery present in a moribund state, there being no time for invasive investigations. Doppler examination in this situation will often provide the diagnosis (such as obstructed mitral prosthesis by showing a very prolonged pressure half-time) and allow appropriate and immediate surgery.

Cardiogenic shock

Whatever the underlying cause, patients with shock have hypoperfusion of vital organs which will result in ischaemia, cellular dysfunction and eventually permanent damage if the process is uncorrected. The situation is often complicated by multisystem failure.

It is essential to make the correct diagnosis of the underlying problem so that appropriate treatment can be given. A patient has the clinical syndrome of shock when there is hypotension associated with poor tissue perfusion. Thus, the patient will usually have a low systolic blood pressure and severely reduced cardiac output manifesting clinically with a cool periphery, often with cyanosis and associated with oliguria or anuria.

The main types of shock must be differentiated as their treatments are very different. Unless treatment is prompt, recovery will not ensue.

1. Cardiogenic (cause is primarily cardiac).
2. Hypovolaemic (reduced circulating blood volume).
3. Septic (bacteraemia).
4. Vasogenic (e.g. anaphylaxis).

Shock due to hypovolaemia is common. The reduction in circulating volume may have many causes and will result in a low JVP and CVP and fluid replacement should commence. Blood or blood products should be given where haemorrhage is the underlying cause but saline or Ringer's solution can be given immediately.

Cardiogenic shock following myocardial infarction may be irreversible if it is associated with extensive myocardial necrosis. However, it can be difficult to know whether impairment of ventricular function following infarction is irreversible. This is particularly true in patients who have received thrombolytic therapy, where recovery of function occurs over several days and even weeks.

Table 1.2 Causes of hypovolaemic shock

	Fluid lost/replacement
Haemorrhage	Blood
Extensive burns Pancreatitis	Plasma

Dehydration or
  inappropriate
  diuretic therapy
Vomiting/diarrhoea
	Saline

Table 1.3 Causes of vasogenic shock

- Anaphylaxis (rare)
Spinal anaesthesia
Drugs
Streptokinase (usually transient)
Reperfusion of right coronary artery (Bezold–Jarisch reflex)

Table 1.4 Causes of cardiogenic shock

Usually requiring medical treatment
    extensive myocardial infarction
    myocardial ischaemia
    myocardial depression after cardiac bypass (may be transient)
    right ventricular infarction
    acute myocarditis
    arrhythmias (usually associated with other cardiac disease)

Usually requiring surgical treatment
    circulatory obstruction e.g. thrombosed prosthetic valve, massive pulmonary
        embolism
    acute valve rupture, papillary muscle rupture post-MI, cusp rupture due to
        endocarditis
    cardiac shunt, e.g. post-infarct VSD

For most patients with cardiogenic shock following myocardial infarction, the immediate question must be whether there is an underlying correctable mechanical problem. Clinical examination may reveal the presence of a new murmur secondary to papillary muscle rupture or ventricular septal defect (VSD), while in the absence of a murmur, cardiac rupture and tamponade should be

Table 1.5 Investigations used in the diagnosis of cardiogenic shock

	Echo	*Doppler*	*Swan–Ganz*
VSD	++	++	+++ (O_2 sat.)
Ruptured papillary muscle	+	++	+ (large v wave)
Tamponade	+++	–	+–
Obstructed prosthesis	++	+++	–
Extensive infarction	++	–	++
Right ventricular infarction	++	–	+++

considered. The key investigation for the latter is echocardiography, while for the former two the diagnosis can be confirmed by combined echo–Doppler investigation or by means of a Swan–Ganz catheter.

Surgical treatment

Early surgical treatment is indicated where there is a surgically correctable lesion, although there is debate about the precise timing in patients with post-infarction VSD. Intra-aortic balloon pumping can be used to support the circulation until surgery is undertaken.

Where no surgical lesion is present, or where there is doubt about the underlying aetiology of the shock, then it is useful to perform measurements of the pulmonary artery wedge pressure. Knowledge of the wedge pressure clearly differentiates between hypovolaemic and cardiogenic shock and helps to clarify the situation in the intermediate situations of right ventricular infarction.

Table 1.6 RA and PAW measurements in various forms of shock

Example	*RA mean pressure* (mmHg)	*PAW mean pressure* (mmHg)	*BP*
Haemorrhage	Low–2	Low–2	70/40
Tamponade	High–25	High–25	65/40
Cardiogenic, e.g. VSD	High–15	High–32	75/50
RV infarct	High–18	Low–6	75/50

Medical treatment

In the absence of a surgically correctable cause and if right ventricular infarction has been excluded, then the prognosis is generally poor. Drug therapy is aimed at optimising haemodynamic parameters, primarily with inotropic support. If the wedge pressure is very high, with resultant pulmonary oedema, then nitrates can be used cautiously. Combinations of 'off-loading' (e.g. sodium nitroprusside) and inotropic agents (e.g. dopamine) are sometimes used with the aim of raising cardiac output, increasing renal blood flow and reducing intrapulmonary pressures. Such therapy requires careful haemodynamic monitoring, ideally by Swan–Ganz catheterisation and arterial monitoring, and urinary catheterisation for hourly urine measurements. If the patient is distressed or in pulmonary oedema then opiates should be given and high-concentration oxygen administered.

Additional measures

Where shock is precipitated by an arrhythmia such as ventricular tachycardia (VT), then DC cardioversion is appropriate.

Where shock is complicated by arrhythmias these may be very difficult to treat. If the rhythm is atrial fibrillation then digoxin should be given. Most agents used for ventricular arrhythmias result in myocardial depression and so should be avoided if possible. Amiodarone can be given but rapid dosing can result in acute hypotension.

Anecdotal cases of successful treatment of post-infarction cardiogenic shock using streptokinase have been reported.

Cardiorespiratory arrest

The sudden arrest of the circulation or of respiration is clearly an extreme medical emergency. It may not be immediately clear which system is primarily responsible for the arrest but cessation of one is inevitably followed by the other and brain death follows if both are not restored within 3–4 minutes.

Respiratory arrest may be due to depression of respiratory drive caused by disease or drugs such as opiates.

Cardiac 'arrest' is mediated by:

- ventricular fibrillation (occasionally rapid VT)
- ventricular standstill or asystole
- electromechanical dissociation (no output despite adequate rhythm).

Cardiac arrest may be precipitated by:

- acute ischaemia or infarction
- hypoxia
- electrolyte imbalance
- acidosis.

Cardiac arrest

In the intensive care situation, the patient will usually be monitored at the time of arrest, making management somewhat easier. In some cases of asystole a single blow to the chest may be sufficient to restore the circulation. If not, then the treatment will depend on the cardiac rhythm. Patients with ventricular fibrillation should have direct current defibrillation as soon as possible. There is good evidence that the success of defibrillation is inversely related to the duration of fibrillation.

It is difficult to give firm guidelines for the management of cardiac arrest as the precise circumstances vary. Some patients with asystole continue to have adequate respiration during the arrest providing the circulation is adequately maintained by massage. In this situation, endotracheal intubation and artificial respiration are not required unless the situation deteriorates.

Given these provisos, it is reasonable to follow the 'ABC' of resuscitation.

A – Airway

Check for any obstruction to the airway and remove it if present. Well-fitting dentures need not be removed. Frequently there will be vomitus which should be removed using suction, if available. Obstruction of the airway by the tongue is prevented by tilting the head back and pulling the angles of the jaw anteriorly.

B – Breathing

If the patient is not breathing adequately, then assistance must be given. The method used will depend on the expertise of those present. Mouth-to-mouth resuscitation can be used if no equipment is available. Usually an Ambu bag and airway will be available. If experienced personnel are present then it is preferable to insert an endotracheal tube.

Whichever method is used, it is important to check that it is effective by noting that the chest rises and falls or by auscultation.

High-concentration oxygen should be administered.

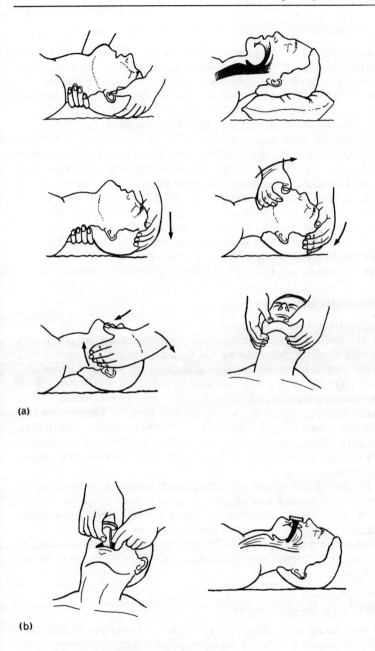

(a)

(b)

Figure 1.1 (a) and (b) Preservation of the airway

C – Circulation

Cardiac massage can provide adequate circulation for prolonged periods providing it is effectively done. For this to be achieved it must be performed on a firm surface, if necessary on the floor. If the arrest is primarily of cardiac origin then massage alone can allow continued delivery of oxygen for about 30 seconds. Frequently, massage and ventilation are required.

Sternal compression is performed at between 80 and 100 beats per minute, moving the sternum 2 inches (5 cm)towards the spine with each compression. Although synchronisation with ventilation is not essential, it is generally easier to synchronise using an agreed regime such as five massages to each ventilation. Success as measured by the normalisation of pupillary size *must* be confirmed and continued. Having established ventilation and circulation, the next step is to make an accurate diagnosis of the cardiac rhythm if this has not already been done. Further measures depend on the type of arrest and will require adequate venous access.

Ventricular fibrillation

Defibrillation with 200 joules will frequently be successful. If not, or if fibrillation is recurrent then a further shock at 200 joules should be given, followed by 400 joules if this is not successful. If these measures are not successful then an i.v. bolus of lignocaine (100 mg) should be given followed by further defibrillation. With increasing time a successful outcome becomes less likely. If it is likely that the patient is severely acidotic then i.v. bicarbonate can be administered but this should not be used routinely. Alternative antiarrhythmic agents can be used if lignocaine is not successful. There is no real limit to the number of times defibrillation can be performed.

In the initial stages of resuscitation there is little point in performing further investigations. After resuscitation the patient must be carefully monitored. Hypokalaemia and hypomagnesaemia predispose to ventricular fibrillation (both of which are common in patients on diuretic therapy). Thus, measurement of electrolytes, particularly potassium and magnesium, may be of value.

Ventricular standstill/asystole

In this situation the priority is to obtain and continue to maintain optimal cardiorespiratory function in an attempt to improve the metabolic status which has resulted in the arrest. If an adequate

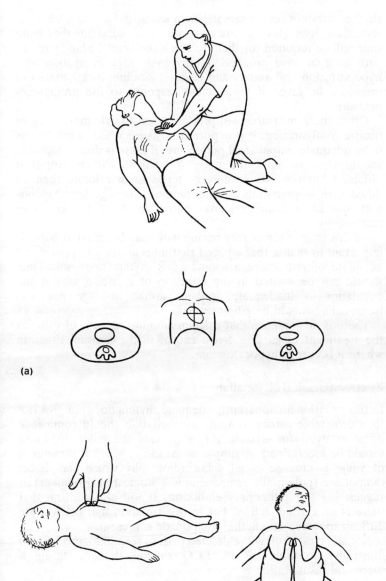

(a)

(b)

Figure 1.2 External cardiac massage (*a*) in the adult; (*b*) in the neonate and infant

rhythm does not return rapidly, then i.v. atropine and adrenaline should be given. (If drugs are given via a peripheral line then more time will be required for them to reach the heart.) Many patients with asystole have progressed through a stage of hypotension, hypoperfusion and anoxia and acidosis. Sodium bicarbonate can therefore be given if there is no response to the preliminary measures.

Often these measures will produce a cardiac rhythm, often of bizarre configuration. It is important to assess whether this results in an adequate output (feel pulse) and, if there is doubt, massage should continue until the pulse is adequate. If an output is obtained but the rate is slow or tends to deteriorate then an infusion of isoprenaline is often helpful. Massage simultaneous with the ECG complexes may allow the heart to take over successfully.

At this stage a temporary pacing wire may be inserted but it is important to realise that a paced rhythm is unlikely to provide an adequate output where a spontaneous rhythm does not. Time should not be wasted in the insertion of a pacing wire if the circulation is inadequate, rather cardiac massage and i.v. isoprenaline should be administered.

There is no evidence that calcium administration is of value in the treatment of cardiac arrest except in the unusual situation where it occurs in hypocalcaemia.

Electromechanical dissociation

In this situation an apparently adequate rhythm does not give rise to a detectable cardiac output. Resuscitation should commence immediately, as for asystole. If time permits, the underlying cause should be ascertained. A simple investigation which is sometimes of value is cross-sectional echocardiography which can detect tamponade (potentially remediable in a surgical environment) or suggest massive pulmonary embolism. It will also confirm that there is no cardiac action, but in this situation it is often more difficult to interpret whether tamponade is present.

Not all arrests follow the defined pattern seen in Figure 1.3. An illustrative example of the ECG rhythm changes during a successful resuscitation is:

(a) ventricular tachycardia – hypotension – rapidly degenerating to:
(b) ventricular tachycardia – no output – 200 J;
(c) bizarre ventricular complexes – cardiac massage;
(d) idioventricular rhythm – good output;

(e) episodes of asystole – massage + adrenaline;
(f) bursts of VT – stabilising to nodal and finally to:
(g) sinus rhythm.

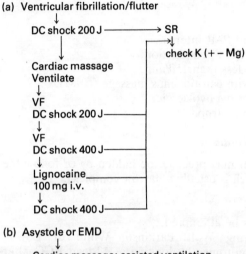

(a) Ventricular fibrillation/flutter

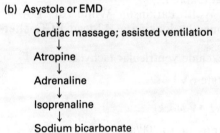

(b) Asystole or EMD

Figure 1.3 Scheme of management of (*a*) ventricular fibrillation/flutter; (*b*) asystole or electromechanical dissociation

Cardiac arrhythmias

Tachycardias

There are two main mechanisms which produce tachycardias but it is seldom possible to determine the mechanism from the surface ECG.

1. *Increased automaticity*. The intrinsic 'firing rate' of a particular specialised myocardial cell when automaticity increases and therefore takes over as the 'pacemaker'.

2. *Re-entry*. A large or small circus movement begins where propagated electrical activity is self-sustaining.

A summary of the common tachycardias and a guide to their identification is given below.

Sinus tachycardia

- Normal P waves and P–R interval.
- 1:1 atrioventricular (AV) conduction.
- Heart rate 'always' less than 150/min.
  May slow slightly with carotid sinus massage (CSM).
- Consider: blood loss/hypovolaemia;
  excessive inotropes.

Supraventricular tachycardia

- P waves present but may precede, be hidden by or follow the QRS complex (which is usually a narrow complex).
- 1:1 AV conduction.
- Heart rate 150–220.
  CSM should always be attempted.
- Consider: underlying Wolff–Parkinson–White or Lown–Ganong–Levine syndromes by looking at 12-lead ECG after return to sinus rhythm.
- If broad complex then exclude ventricular tachycardia (VT).

Atrial lines may precipitate SVT.

Atrial tachycardia (usually 2:1 AV block)

- P waves present (frequently up to 300/min) seen best in V_1.
- 2:1 AV conduction (associated ventricular rate 150/min).
- CSM often increases AV block transiently.

Atrial flutter

- F (flutter) waves present – broad sawtooth atrial waves (rate about 300/min).
- CSM transiently increases AV block.

Atrial fibrillation

- Absent P waves – fibrillary waves may be seen.
- Ventricular complexes irregular – often rapid in cases of recent onset (130–200/min).
- CSM slows ventricular rate.

Ventricular tachycardia

- P waves present but may not be obvious (normal 'sinus' rate).
- Total dissociation between atrial and ventricular activity (unless retrograde VA conduction).
- Ventricular rate between 120–300.
- QRS complexes broad.
- R–R interval may be very slightly irregular.
- CSM usually has no effect.
- Consider: hypokalaemia;
  drugs (including anti-arrhythmic agents and inotropes);
  Swan–Ganz can precipitate.

Ventricular fibrillation

- Chaotic rhythm.
- Seldom self-terminating unless torsade de pointes.

Torsade de pointes

- Bursts of bizarre rhythm similar to VF.
- Recurrent self-terminating episodes.
  Consider: long QT syndrome/hypokalaemia.

Differentiation between ventricular and supraventricular origin of a broad complex tachycardia

This confusion arises because in some cases of supraventricular tachycardia (SVT) there is aberrant conduction of the impulse giving a bundle branch pattern (broad QRS). However, one of the commonest mistakes in the management of cardiac arrhythmias results from the overdiagnosis of aberrant conduction and therefore misinterpretation of ventricular tachycardia (VT) as being of SV origin.

The following points are helpful in differentiating between SVT and VT. A 12-lead ECG is essential for accurate diagnosis.

1. Look for AV dissociation. If P waves are seen moving irregularly and independently through the QRS complexes, then the diagnosis must be that of VT.
2. If the QRS duration is greater than 0.14 seconds, VT should be diagnosed.
3. Previous ECGs are of great help. A change in direction of electrical activity suggests VT.

4. The presence of fusion beats indicates VT. These are occasional sinus beats which manage to 'capture' producing antegrade conduction and are then met by the ventricular complex travelling in the reverse direction. This usually results in a slightly narrower complex than those of the VT beats.

Bradycardias

Bradycardias fall into two main categories:

1. Those which result in a reduction in the sinus (pacemaker) rate.
2. Those which result in bradycardia due to block in the conducting system beyond the sinus node.

Sinus arrest

Here the sinus node fails to produce an impulse for a variable period of time. If the sinus node fails to produce an impulse for a prolonged period of time then an 'escape rhythm' may occur but sometimes asystole persists. Escape rhythms tend to be of a slower rate the further down the conducting system they arise.

Paradoxically, profound bradycardias may be responsible for precipitating ventricular tachycardia in some cases by allowing expression of ventricular impulses.

Sino-atrial exit block

This is similar to sinus arrest in that no P wave appears to the ECG but it is caused by block to the conduction of a normal sinus node impulse. The pause seen in the ECG is therefore a multiple of the normal PP interval.

AV block

1. *1st degree* heart block does not result in bradycardia. It does not require treatment.
2. *2nd degree – Wenckebach*. Progressive prolongation of the PR interval occurs until finally the P wave does not conduct through the AV node. The heart rate is seldom slow and although the pulse will be slightly irregular, symptoms do not occur. No treatment is required unless the block progresses.
3. *2nd degree – Möbitz (type II)*. Although the PR interval is normal for those beats which are conducted, in 2nd degree Möbitz block other atrial impulses are blocked at the AV node.

Commonly, every second P wave is not conducted but, depending on the clinical situation, other more serious bradycardias may supervene. If symptoms occur or there is haemodynamic disturbance then treatment is indicated.
4. *3rd degree (complete heart block; CHB).* A major feature of CHB is complete dissociation between atrial and ventricular activity. However, it is important to realise that AV dissociation is not synonymous with CHB.

Complete heart block

Atrial impulses produced at the normal rate do not progress beyond the AV node. The ventricular rate depends on the site within the conducting system below the AV node which takes over as the effective pacemaker. If the origin of the ventricular rhythm is lower down the ventricle, the heart rate is likely to be slower, the QRS complex broader and the rhythm generally less stable.

Complete heart block may be due to: surgery – aortic, mitral and especially tricuspid valve replacement; ischaemia/infarction; conducting system fibrosis (with increasing age); or it may be congenital.

AV dissociation

The atrial rate is normal or slow but there is dissociation between it and the ventricles because the ventricular rate is a little faster than the atrial rate. The site of origin of the ventricular impulse is usually close to the AV node so that the QRS complex remains quite narrow. There is no bradycardia and no treatment is required. (Also note that a form of AV dissociation occurs in VT.)

Anti-arrhythmic drugs

CLASS I. Membrane stabilizing (Reduce conductivity, excitability and automaticity.)

Subgroup Ia – moderate reduction in conductivity and prolongation of action potential duration.

1. Quinidine
   - Indications: ventricular arrhythmias.
   - Dose by mouth: 200–400 mg 3–4 times daily.
   - Side-effects: diarrhoea, thrombocytopenia, haemolytic anaemia. Also prolongs the QT interval and may lead to torsade de pointes.
   - Contraindications: heart block.

2. Procainamide
   - Indications: ventricular and supraventricular arrhythmias.
   - Dose: by mouth: 250 mgs 4–6 times daily.
         i.v. injection: 25–350 mg/min, max: 1 g
   - Side-effects: diarrhoea, fever, lupus erythematosus-like syndrome, QT interval prolongation.
   - Contraindications: heart block, heart failure.

3. Disopyramide
   - Indications: post-MI ventricular arrhythmias, supraventricular arrhythmias.
   - Dose: by mouth: 300–800 mg daily.
         i.v. injection: 2 mg/kg over 5 min followed by oral dose 200 mg.
         i.v. infusion: 400 µg/kg/h to max 800 mg daily.
   - Side-effects: hypotension, severe anticholinergic effects, QT interval prolongation.
   - Contraindications: heart block, heart failure, glaucoma.

Subgroup Ib – Depression of automaticity, reduction of amplitude or delayed after-depolarisation with increased VF threshold.

1. Lignocaine
   - Indications: ventricular ectopics – more than 8/min, multifocal, runs of VT. Ectopic on T wave, haemodynamic impairment.
   - Dose: 1 mg/kg initial dose, followed by infusion of 1–4 mg/min.
   - Side-effects: CNS signs (convulsions).
   - Contraindications: liver failure, severe low cardiac output, heart block.

2. Mexiletine
   - Indications: ventricular arrhythmias.
   - Dose: by mouth 400 mg initially followed by 200 mg after 2 hours and 3–4 times daily.
         i.v. injection: 25 mg/min for 5–10 min, followed by infusion of 250 mg/hour for 1 hour and 125 mg for 2 hours.
   - Contraindications: heart block.

3. Tocainide
   - Indications: severe and refractory ventricular arrhythmias.
   - Dose: by mouth: 400 mg 3 times a day.
         i.v. injection: 500 mg over 30 min followed by oral dose.
   - Side-effects: CNS signs, nausea, aplastic anaemia, fibrosing alveolitis.
   - Contraindications: severe renal or hepatic failure, heart failure.

4. Phenytoin
   - Indications: digitalis-induced arrhythmias.
   - Dose: by mouth: 300–400 mg/day.
             i.v. injection: 3–5 mg/kg over 10 min.
   - Side-effects: CNS symptoms, hypotension.
   - Contraindications: SVT, heart block.

Subgroup Ic – Do not prolong ventricular repolarization period.
Prolong QRS.

1. Flecainide
   - Indications: ventricular arrhythmias.
   - Dose: by mouth: 100–200 mg 12-hourly.
             i.v. injection: 2 mg/kg over 30 min.
             i.v. infusion: 250 µg/kg/h.
   - Side-effects: nausea, dizziness.
   - Contraindications: heart failure, heart block.

2. Encainide

3. Lorcainide

CLASS II. Beta blockers

1. Beta-1 selective: Acebutolol
                         Atenolol
                         Metoprolol
2. Non-selective: Propranolol
                         Oxprenolol
                         Sotalol
                         Nadolol
                         Timolol
                         Pindolol
3. Beta and alpha effects: Labetalol

CLASS III. Repolarization prolongers

1. Amiodarone
   - Indications: WPW syndrome, refractory supraventricular and ventricular arrhythmias.
   - Dose: by mouth: 200 mg 8-hourly for one week, followed by 200 mg 12-hourly for one week and then 200 mg daily.
             i.v. injection: 5 mg/kg over 1–2 hours, then 1 g over 24 hours.
   - Side-effects: neuropathy, thyroid dysfunction, hepatitis, CNS signs, corneal microdeposits, photosensitivity.
   - Contraindications: heart block, pregnancy.

2. Bretylium
   - Indications: refractory ventricular arrhythmias.
   - Dose: i.m. injection: 5 mg/kg 1 dose.
            i.v. injection: 5–10 mg/kg over 10 min.
            infusion: 1–2 mg/min.
   - Side-effects: nausea, hypotension.

CLASS IV. Calcium antagonists

1. Verapamil
   - Indications: supraventricular tachyarrhythmias.
   - Dose: by mouth: 40–120 mg 8-hourly.
            i.v. injection: 5–10 mg over 5–10 min.
   - Side-effects: vomiting, bradycardia, hypotension.
   - Contraindications: heart block, heart failure.

2. Diltiazem

PACING: over or underdrive or programmed electrical stimuli

May terminate techycardias.

Pacemakers

The increasing use and complexity of pacing systems means that an understanding of currently available pacemakers is desirable.

All pacemakers consist of three main components.

1. *Power supply* for electrical energy.
2. *Electronic circuitry* for sensing cardiac electrical activity and controlling pacing output.
3. *Electrode (lead)* for transmitting electrical signals from and to the heart.

If pacing is required for a short period then an external generator (temporary pacing box) is used. It is usually connected to the right ventricle (endocardial pacing) by a transvenous pacing electrode with a positive and negative electrode close to the tip (bipolar system). During cardiac operations, thin pacing wires may also be attached to the myocardial surface (epicardial pacing) and externalised to allow temporary pacing. Temporary pacing may also be achieved by oesophageal pacing or external stimulation in the emergency situation.

If pacing is required long-term, then a small permanent system is implanted. These pacemakers can be of either the above bipolar or of unipolar type. Unipolar systems use the casing of the pulse generator to complete the electrical circuit.

Endocardial systems are commonly placed in the prepectoral region, with the pacing electrode entering the venous system via the cephalic or subclavian vein. Local anaesthesia, light sedation (diazepam 10 mg orally) and antibiotic prophylaxis are usually all that is required.

Epicardial systems require a thoracotomy for lead placement, the generator being sited in the abdominal wall.

Pacing systems

A three figure pacing code is used to describe the pacing function of individual systems.

- First letter: describes the chamber(s) paced.
- Second letter: describes the chamber(s) sensed.
- Third letter: describes the pacing mode in response to sensed activity: I = inhibition, T = trigger.

The second and third letters can be indicated as 'O' if the sections are not applicable, i.e. VOO – ventricular fixed rate pacing with no sensing function.

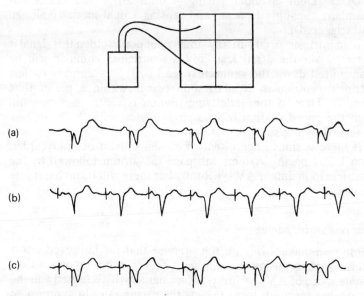

(a)

(b)

(c)

Figure 1.4 Dual chamber pacing: (*a*) atrial sense → ventricular pacing; (*b*) atrial pace → normal AV conduction → ventricular sense; (*c*) atrial pace → ventricular pace

VVI (ventricle paced, ventricle sensed, inhibited mode)

The commonest form of pacing. Only the ventricle is paced and so there is no AV synchrony. Intrinsic ventricular electrical activity is sensed, resulting in inhibition of pacing output. Thus if AV conduction is restored and/or the heart rate is adequate then the intrinsic cardiac rhythm will express itself. This prevents the possibility of a pacing impulse landing on the upstroke of the T wave with the associated risk of inducing ventricular fibrillation.

AAI (atrium paced, atrium sensed, inhibited mode)

Infrequently used but the optimum pacing mode in some patients with sinus-node disease (e.g. sinus arrest in sick-sinus syndrome). For atrial pacing to be employed safely it is essential that AV conduction is normal (confirm by pacing the atria at 120/min).

Physiological pacing

True physiological pacing implies the ability to increase heart rate in response to exercise and the maintenance of AV synchrony.

DDD [Dual chamber pacing – both atrial and ventricular chambers capable of pacing and sensing – dual mode (inhibited and triggered)].

If an intrinsic atrial (usually sinus) beat occurs, then this signal is detected via the atrial lead and a ventricular stimulus will be transmitted down the ventricular lead by the pacemaker (unless intrinsic ventricular depolarisation occurs within a preset time period). Thus, if the underlying rhythm is ventricular standstill then the paced rhythm will be physiological with the heart rate governed by the sinus node rate.

If there is sinus node disease with sinus arrest or bradycardia, then DDD pacing systems will pace the atrium followed by the ventricle to maintain AV synchrony but there will be no heart rate variability.

Rate responsive pacing

These pacemakers rely on the premise that for improved effort tolerance then the increase in heart rate is more important than maintenance of AV synchrony. Muscular activity is sensed and the pacemaker responds by increasing the pacing rate. In appropriate cases, either the ventricle or atrium can be paced but the former is much more common.

Programmability

Most implanted systems nowadays are programmable using an external radiofrequency transmitter. Parameters which can be altered include rate, voltage, pulse width, sensitivity, pacing mode, hysteresis and, in dual chambered systems, the AV delay.

The nomenclature for programmable functions is:

P = simple programmable (rate or output)
M = multi-programmable
C = communicating (telemetry)
O = none

Anti-tachycardia pacing

These systems are capable of detecting atrial tachyarrhythmias and use electrical stimulation to terminate the tachycardia.

The nomenclature for special anti-tachycardia functions is:

B = burst
N = normal
S = scanning
E = external

Implantable defibrillators

In a few patients recurrent ventricular fibrillation occurs which is not prevented by drug therapy. An implanted device can detect VF and provide sufficient electrical energy for defibrillation via a pad sewn on to the epicardial surface of the heart.

Indications for permanent pacing

1. Symptomatic complete heart block (non-infarction).
2. Complete heart block *which does not recover:*
   (a) after myocardial infarction (wait two weeks);
   (b) after valve replacement – particularly tricuspid – also mitral and aortic (wait up to one week);
   (c) after CABG – as for myocardial infarction.
3. Bifascicular block or bundle branch block with transient 2nd or 3rd degree block after anterior myocardial infarction.
4. Symptomatic sinus arrest or AV block (non-infarction):
   (a) if not drug related;
   (b) if caused by drugs which are necessary to control concomitant tachycardias.

Pacing problems

Bradycardia (Figure 1.5)

1. No pacing spike.
   - Caused by: lead break/connection problem resulting in no current reaching the myocardium; or inappropriate sensing of electrical (interference) or mechanical signals (myoinhibition) or generator failure.
   - Remedy: check connections (if temporary system); check for evidence of interference.
2. Pacing spike but no capture.
   - Caused by: increased threshold or lead displacement/ fracture.
   - Remedy: increase pacing output or reposition lead.
3. Failure to sense: results in inappropriate pacing spikes. The intrinsic rhythm not sensed and therefore pacing output is not inhibited. Some pacing spikes will capture but others will fall within the refractory period. In patients with ischaemic heart disease this may produce ventricular fibrillation.
   - Remedy: increase sensitivity (so that small signals are detected) or reposition lead.

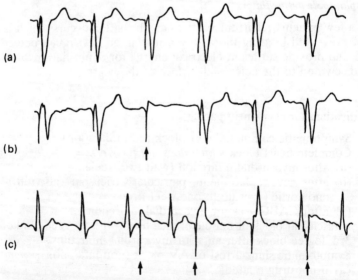

(a)

(b)

(c)

Figure 1.5 Ventricular pacing (VVI): (*a*) normal pacing; (*b*) intermittent failure to capture; (*c*) intermittent failure to sense

Tachycardia

Usually not pacing-related but secondary to underlying disease. May be pacemaker-mediated tachycardia with DDD pacing (ventricular pacing results in retrograde conduction up bundle of His and activation of the atria; this atrial activity is sensed, thereby triggering a ventricular pacing impulse which sets up an artificial 'circus' tachycardia).

Hypotension/dizziness/breathlessness (pacemaker syndrome)

A small number of patients are very sensitive to ventricular pacing. This usually occurs only if there is retrograde conduction and the resulting increase in atrial pressures stimulates reflex hypotension. The constellation of symptoms this may produce is termed the 'pacemaker syndrome'.

Technical aspects of pacing

Patients returning from cardiac surgery often have temporary pacing systems in place and these may either be single (atrial or ventricular) or dual (atrial and ventricular) chamber systems. The number of problems which may arise is obviously increased with a dual chamber system and it is essential to understand the basic principles of pacing before attempting to rectify a malfunctioning system.

Single chamber pacemakers

Single chamber, temporary external pacemakers usually have just two or three controls which allow easy adjustment by the operator to suit the needs of the patient.

1. *Rate control:* typically in the range 30–130 p.p.m. but some have optional high rate mode for simple tachycardia control by overdrive pacing.
2. *Output control:* either graduated in volts or milliamps. By slowly reducing the output level, the minimum energy required to cause depolarisation of the myocardium can be determined. The figure obtained is the voltage or current threshold and will give an indication of the effectiveness of the lead attachment to the epicardium. The final setting of the output control should be high enough to allow for deterioration of the lead/epicardial interface without loss of capture, i.e. if the threshold is 1 v, then set pacemaker to 4 v. Temporary epicardial systems can be

unstable and threshold levels should be checked at regular intervals. Atrial systems in particular are prone to problems, especially sensing ones.
3. *Sensitivity control.* The standard mode of operation of a temporary pacemaker is that of demand pacing. That is, the pacemaker will discharge an output pulse if the patient's rate falls below the setting of the rate control and will cease to discharge a pulse when the patient's heart rate exceeds the rate control setting. For this on-demand function to work effectively, the pacemaker must be able to detect the patient's cardiac activity via the pacing leads. The epicardial electrogram must be of sufficient amplitude for the pacemaker to sense it and revert to its stand-by mode. Some pacemakers have an adjustable sensitivity control to allow the detection of small signals. It should be realised that making a pacemaker more sensitive will also increase the possibility of interference by non-cardiac signals. Making the control less sensitive will increase the possibility of the pacemaker discharging inappropriately during normal heart activity.

Dual chamber pacemakers

To create a more physiological pacing action, there is an increasing use of dual chamber units which are able to pace and sense activity from both atria and ventricles.

In addition to the rate control, there will be two output controls and two sensitivity controls for atrial and ventricular adjustment. Atrial epicardial signals are generally much lower in amplitude than are ventricular ones and the atrial sensitivity control will have a lower range setting than the ventricular one. (Loss of atrial sensing and pacing is one of the most common problems in temporary dual chamber pacing systems.) Probably the only extra facility will be the AV delay.

AV delay control

This is to vary the time between the generation of a pulse and the sensing of spontaneous activity in the atrial or the ventricular channel. The range of adjustment is in the order of 50–250 ms.

General points

By adjustment of the controls it is possible to obtain a number of options, depending on the particular patient's underlying rhythm and requirements. These can be summarised as follows:

1. Sense atrium – sense ventricle.
2. Sense atrium – pace ventricle.
3. Pace atrium – sense ventricle.
4. Pace atrium – pace ventricle.

Adjustment of the AV delay control can allow normal AV nodal conduction, where this exists, and thus obviate the need to pace the ventricles.

The classification of the systems is the same as that for implanted pacemakers. The standard ventricular demand pacemaker will be coded as VVI, an atrial demand system will be AAI and a complete dual chamber system will be DDD.

Heart failure

Left heart failure

Left heart failure may develop in a wide variety of cardiac diseases which can be grouped according to the mechanism by which they are produced.

1. Increased afterload:
   (a) aortic stenosis;
   (b) sub-aortic stenosis;
   (c) aortic coarctation;
   (d) hypertension.
2. Increased volume load:
   (a) aortic regurgitation;
   (b) mitral regurgitation;
   (c) hyperthyroidism (multiple mechanism);
   (d) Paget's disease;
   (e) arteriovenous fistula.
3. Decreased myocardial contractility:
   (a) myocardial infarction;
   (b) severe myocardial ischaemia;
   (c) dilated cardiomyopathy;
   (d) acute myocarditis;
   (e) Beriberi.
4. Mitral valve obstruction

Whatever the cause of the heart failure, the end result is a rise in left atrial and pulmonary venous pressure. This is responsible for the classical symptoms of dyspnoea, orthopnoea, and paroxysmal nocturnal dyspnoea, and pulmonary oedema.

The associated *clinical features* which are commonly present are:

- tachycardia
- pulsus alternans
- displaced apex beat
- triple rhythm
- basal crepitations.

Radiological features of left heart failure or pulmonary oedema will usually be present:

- upper lobe venous distension
- pleural effusions
- Kerley 'B' lines
- fluffy shadowing, often of 'batswing' appearance but may extend more peripherally or even be unilateral.

Medical treatment

The treatment of heart failure should be directed at the underlying cause or mechanism. Although in many cases this will mean surgical treatment, initial medical therapy to control the heart failure will be required:

1. High concentrations of oxygen.
2. Opiate.
3. Intravenous diuretics.
4. Digoxin if the rhythm is atrial fibrillation (+ rapid rate).
5. Afterload reduction if hypertensive (e.g. hydralazine).
6. Preload reduction for pulmonary oedema (e.g. nitrates).
7. Inotropes if reduced contractility.
8. If pulmonary oedema does not respond to the above measures then ventilation should be considered.

Surgical treatment

In *aortic stenosis* the onset of heart failure is an indication that surgery is indicated. In *mitral stenosis*, heart failure may be controlled for many years before operation is needed but in some situations, such as pregnancy, urgent valvotomy is required. Acute *aortic* or *mitral regurgitation*, such as may occur with endocarditis, may also need urgent valve replacement. Surgery for heart failure secondary to *ischaemic heart disease* is generally less successful; failure following *myocardial infarction* resulting in a large segment of myocardial akinesia is not amenable to surgery. If, however, there is a dyskinetic area (*aneurysm*) then resection may improve the haemodynamic situation. Surgery is indicated for heart failure due to transient *myocardial ischaemia* which will respond to myocardial revascularisation.

Treatment of chronic heart failure

Secondary compensatory mechanisms result in peripheral vaso-constriction (increased afterload), partly mediated by stimulation of the renin–angiotensin system which also results in sodium and water retention. Drug therapy:

1. *Diuretics.* Loop diuretics such as bumetamide or frusemide are still a corner-stone of treatment. It is sometimes helpful to add a thiazide in cases which are resistant. Aldosterone antagonists are helpful in counteracting secondary fluid retention and conserve potassium.
2. *Vasodilators.* The advent of angiotensin converting enzyme (ACE) inhibitors has been a major development in the treatment of cardiac failure. They not only result in haemody-namic and symptomatic improvement but also improve prognosis. They must be used with caution. Profound hypotension can occur, particularly in patients who are on large doses of diuretics. In patients with renal impairment frequent monitoring of electrolytes is required as further renal deterioration may occur. Because they inhibit the renin–angiotensin system, aldosterone antagonists (and/or potassium supplements) are usually not required. If ACE inhibition cannot be tolerated, an alternative approach to vasodilator therapy is to use a combination of afterload reduction (hydralazine) and preload reduction (nitrates).

Right heart failure

Right heart failure is a frequent accompaniment of long-standing left heart failure (which causes pulmonary hypertension). Long-standing pulmonary hypertension of whatever cause will result in right ventricular hypertrophy and eventually in right heart failure.

1. Mediated by pulmonary hypertension:
   (a) primary pulmonary hypertension;
   (b) secondary pulmonary hypertension due to chronic obstructive airways disease, left heart failure, multiple pulmonary emboli, atrial and ventricular septal defects.
2. Mediated by valvular disease:
   (a) pulmonary stenosis (rarely regurgitation);
   (b) tricuspid stenosis or regurgitation.

The *clinical features* of right heart failure are:

- elevated jugular venous pressure
- peripheral oedema
- hepatic congestion
- right ventricular lift
- loud second heart sound (in pulmonary hypertension)
- tricuspid regurgitation
- (pulmonary disease).

Treatment

The treatment of right heart failure should also be directed at correcting the underlying problem, if possible. With right heart failure secondary to pulmonary hypertension, surgical treatment may be too late to reverse the pulmonary vascular changes. Thus if atrial or ventricular septal defects are of sufficient size and are uncorrected then the increased pulmonary blood flow eventually results in irreversible pulmonary hypertension and reversal of shunting from right to left (Eisenmenger's syndrome).

Drug therapy of right heart failure is similar to that for left heart failure.

Ischaemic heart disease

Myocardial ischaemia can be defined as inadequate myocardial perfusion for a given workload. In ischaemic heart disease (IHD) it is due to fixed or variable coronary arterial narrowing. If ischaemia is prolonged, usually because of total coronary occlusion, then myocardial infarction (necrosis) occurs.

Myocardial ischaemia also occurs in the absence of coronary artery disease, particularly in severe aortic stenosis, aortic regurgitation or mitral stenosis.

Four risk factors for IHD can be modified:

1. Smoking.
2. Obesity or excessive fat intake, with resultant hypercholesterolaemia or hyperlipidaemia.
3. Salt ingestion resulting in hypertension.
4. Lack of strenuous exercise.

Other risk factors which are associated with IHD but which cannot be modified are family history, increasing age and diabetes mellitus (genuine insulin-dependent, as opposed to obesity-induced).

Presentation

IHD may present in a variety of ways and thereafter there may be movement from one end of the spectrum to the other.

1. *Sudden death:* ischaemia induces VF or electromechanical dissociation
2. *Myocardial infarction:*
    (a) *transmural* – usually due to *thrombotic* coronary occlusion;
    (b) *non-transmural* – often a tightly stenosed but patent artery is found at coronary angiography (*thrombus* common).
3. *Unstable angina:* pain at rest, usually with ST changes and frequently associated with complex coronary lesions and *thrombus.*
4. *Stable angina:* angina on exertion – usually due to a fixed coronary obstruction.
5. *Vasospastic angina:* acute ischaemia due to coronary spasm, usually with at least some underlying atheroma.
6. *Silent ischaemia:* asymptomatic ischaemia at rest or on exertion associated with ST changes. Episodes of both symptomatic and silent ischaemia may occur in the same patient at different times.

Patients resuscitated from 'sudden death'–generally 'out-of-hospital cardiac arrest'–will usually have had ventricular fibrillation. If there is no rise in cardiac enzymes then these patients are at risk of further life-threatening ischaemic events. Coronary angiography should usually be performed to define the coronary anatomy. If there is clear evidence of myocardial infarction then late recurrence of VF is much less likely.

Myocardial infarction

Presentation

Usually with prolonged, typical (or near-typical) ischaemic pain. Infarction may be asymptomatic or become manifest only when complications arise.

Serious arrhythmias, particularly ventricular fibrillation (VF), occur frequently in the early stages of infarction, particularly within the first hour, in both inferior and anterior infarction. After the second hour the incidence of serious arrhythmias greatly declines. Early (or primary) VF is treated with defibrillation; anti-arrhythmic therapy is not required unless VF is resistant.

Inferior infarction

The parasympathetic nervous system predominates and in the early stages bradycardia and hypotension and nausea are common. Although second degree and complete heartblock are common, normal conduction almost always recovers within two weeks (and usually within a day or two). Prognosis is better than with anterior infarction.

Anterior infarction

The sympathetic system predominates. Left ventricular function is affected to a much greater degree than is usual with inferior infarction. Sinus tachycardia is frequent. It may be indicative of left ventricular failure, which is common. Prognosis is largely dependent on the degree of residual left ventricular function.

Confirmation of the diagnosis of infarction

Early diagnosis is important to allow appropriate intervention (see below). The 12-lead ECG is of paramount importance. It may confirm the diagnosis and indicate the site of infarction. The earliest sign of infarction is localised ST elevation which can occur within 45 seconds of coronary occlusion. (In a few patients the ECG may remain normal for several hours.) As infarction proceeds, there is development of Q waves with loss of R waves in the affected leads.

Serial cardiac enzyme estimations are useful for subsequent confirmation of infarction and give some guide to:

1. Approximate infarct size (area under curve).
2. Whether reperfusion has occurred (early peaking).
3. Whether reocclusion occurs (secondary rise).
4. Whether perioperative myocardial infarction has occurred.

Currently available cardiac enzymes are of little or no value in making an early diagnosis to guide therapy in myocardial infarction because the rise occurs too late. The earliest enzyme to rise is the creatinine kinase and this does not begin until after about four hours. Specific myocardial isoenzyme estimations (CK-MB or LD1) are available which exclude a non-cardiac cause for any increase in total creatine kinase or lactic dehydrogenase.

A peak level of CK within 16 hours of the onset of pain indicates either perfusion of an occluded artery or persistent patency of a severely stenosed, infarct-related artery.

Management of acute myocardial infarction

1. *Pain relief.* Intravenous opiate should be given if pain is present. A trial of glyceryl trinitrin can be given if there is doubt as to whether pain is due to angina or infarction. In about 5% of cases of infarction, coronary spasm plays a predominant role and reperfusion may follow nitrate therapy.
2. *Thrombolytic therapy.* Patients seen early after the onset of infarction should be treated with thrombolytic therapy unless a contraindication exists. Time limits and the optimal agent are changing. The earlier therapy is given, the greater the myocardial salvage. Anterior infarcts up to six hours after the onset of pain, and inferior infarcts up to three hours, should benefit from streptokinase or APSAC; rtPA is much more expensive but is non-antigenic. Recovery of LV function may take two weeks. Reocclusion occurs in about 20% of those with reperfusion; anticoagulants probably reduce the incidence of reocclusion. The role and timing of PTCA following thrombolysis has not yet been clearly defined.
3. *Aspirin.* 300 mg (soluble), then 75 mg (slow-release) twice weekly.
4. *Bed rest, monitoring and early mobilisation.* The period of bed rest has been dramatically cut but during the first 24 hours patients should still be confined to bed and monitored for arrhythmias. They may be allowed to sit in a chair on the second day if all is well and thereafter mobilisation begins.
5. Further management is directed towards the treatment of complications of infarction and prevention of further infarction.

Infective endocarditis

In this intravascular and disseminated form of infection the most common microorganisms isolated are: *Streptococcus viridans* (40–50%); *Streptococcus B* (10–20%); *Staphylococcus aureus* (10–15%); *Staphylococcus epidermidis* (5–10%); Gram-negative bacilli (6–8%); negative cultures (8–12%).

In cases of infective endocarditis of prosthetic valves, the frequency changes to *Streptococci, Staphylococcus aureus,* Gram-negative bacilli and uncommon microorganisms like *Candida*.

The immune system is affected with circulating immune complexes, low complement levels and hyperimmunoglobulinaemia.

There are two clinical phases: one of acute endocarditis with embolic manifestations and low level of circulating immune complexes, and a chronic one with high levels of circulating immune complexes. The most important prognostic factors are: mode of onset, duration of illness, infecting microorganisms, renal complications, CNS complications, haemodynamic deterioration and positivity of cultures after treatment.

Presentation may be with heart failure, sepsis or peripheral embolism, plus signs of aortic or mitral incompetence in the presence of cutaneous signs, glomerulonephritis and/or mycotic aneurysms. In cases of tricuspid involvement (in drug addicts or immunocompromised patients), the septic signs along with lung infiltrates suggest the diagnosis. Prosthetic endocarditis, usually after dental or surgical procedures without antibiotic coverage, presents with signs of prosthetic valvular leakage demonstrated by echo.

Treatment includes specific antibiotics, medications for heart failure, treatment for complications and surgery.

Operation is indicated by haemodynamic deterioration, valve failure, persistent sepsis, systemic embolism and uncommon microorganisms.

Antibiotic prophylaxis

Standard regimen for dental surgery under local anaesthesia

3 g amoxycillin orally as a single dose one hour before the procedure (<10 years, half adult dose; <5 years, quarter adult dose).

Standard regimen for patients allergic to penicillin or who have received penicillin in the previous month

1.5 g oral erythromycin 1 h before procedure plus one dose of 0.5 g six hours later (<10 years, half adult dose; <5 years, quarter adult dose).

Dental surgery under general anaesthetic

1 g amoxycillin i.m. (dissolved in 2.5 ml 1% lignocaine) before induction plus one dose of 500 mg orally six hours later (<10 years, half adult dose; <5 years, quarter adult dose).

Procedures other than dental surgery

These include, for example, tonsillectomy/adenoidectomy, abdominal surgery, genito-urinary surgery or instrumentation, drainage of infected tissues. Detailed recommendations are available (British Society of Antimicrobial Therapy, 1982).

High-risk patients

1. Prosthetic valves.
2. Previous bacterial endocarditis.
3. Needing general anaesthesia and allergic to penicillin or having taken penicillin recently.

Detailed recommendations are available (British Society for Antimicrobial Therapy, 1982).

Nursing care

Heart failure

The nurse's rôle in the management of heart failure can be divided into three main categories: detection of complications, administration of drugs and evaluation of treatment.

Observation

Vital signs, properly documented, are a baseline for further observations. Pallor, sweating, cool extremities, the coughing of pink froth, are instantly apparent disaster signs. The recording of intake and output is essential, not only to assess fluid balance but the response to drug therapy. Arrhythmias may be associated with hypoxia, electrolyte disturbances or drug therapy. They are reported immediately.

Care

The patient is nursed in the position most comfortable to him: this is usually a sitting position (semi-Fowler) in bed but occasionally a patient may prefer to be sitting in a large armchair. Any sacral or peripheral oedema should be reported. He should receive a daily bed bath. Frequent washes should be offered if the patient is very sweaty. Some patients may request a fan.

The patient in failure may be extremely frightened for his life; reassurance and sedatives as prescribed will alleviate the stress. All procedures, including the need for cannulae, blood sampling and drug therapy, should be explained to the patient and the relatives.

Cardiac arrhythmias

The nurse's rôle in the management of the patient with cardiac arrhythmias is to detect, record and report arrhythmias and instigate emergency treatment.

Monitoring

Careful shaving without abrasion minimises any irritation from the electrodes. The leads of the monitor are attached and the alarms are set, the usual range of rate being 50–150/min, outside which an alarm is triggered which will also lead to a 'write-out' at the central console.

In progressive coronary care units and medical wards telemetric monitoring may be used. The electrodes are positioned in the usual way and connected to a battery transmitter. Radio signals are received by the central console and the ECG displayed on the screen.

The vital signs are recorded. The skin is frequently observed for changes in colour, temperature and perfusion. The relation between arrhythmia/chest pain is important.

The side-effects of anti-arrhythmic drugs must be known by the nurse in order to detect them (see p. 21).

Cardiac arrest

This may occur at any time. If ventricular fibrillation or tachycardia is associated with unconsciousness, cardioversion should be used. Impregnated jelly pads are placed in position on the patient's chest to prevent burns, and defibrillation is carried out only by experienced personnel, including nursing staff who have extended their rôle.

Synchronised electrocardioversion is used to convert atrial fibrillation and supraventricular tachycardias into sinus rhythm in those patients in whom the arrhythmia, although not usually life threatening, is causing haemodynamic impairment.

Every nurse must be familiar with emergency equipment including defibrillators and know how to switch on, select the energy and charge. They should also be aware of the risks, including those to personnel. Routine checks of this and anaesthetic equipment and drugs are important.

Transvenous pacing

Pacing may be indicated for disturbances of conduction arising from acute myocardial infarction or for chronic irreversible block.

The latter requires a permanent pacing system; the conduction disturbance associated with myocardial infarction is usually (not always) transient.

The patient should be helped to understand the need for the procedure, the technique used and the equipment. A consent form may be signed. The approach will be by the antecubital fossa, femoral or subclavian route.

Assistance, emergency drugs and the defibrillator are provided, and the nurse should observe the monitor for arrhythmias. The nurse should be familiar with the pacemaker system and be able to identify any problems, such as loss of capture and failing to sense. The pacing wire may perforate the right ventricle, which may stimulate muscular twitches of the chest wall; a chest X-ray will confirm the position of the wire. The wound should be dressed as necessary and observed for infection and thrombophlebitis.

Electrodes

Pacing wires are normally identified by the number of electrodes incorporated in the tip of the catheter. A single electrode, a unipolar catheter, requires a second contact to complete the circuit. The bipolar catheter (two poles), is preferred. Quadripolar and hexipolar catheters may also be used for electrophysiology studies and multichamber pacing.

The pulse generator

This is battery operated and transmits electrical impulses down the electrode to the heart. In temporary pacing the generator is external; in permanent systems it is implanted.

Insertion of temporary pacing electrode

Using an aseptic technique, the skin is prepared and a local anaesthetic infiltrated. An introducer is positioned in the selected vein and the pacing electrode introduced and advanced into the superior vena cava, to the right atrium, tricuspid valve and into the right ventricle, under fluoroscopy. Once in position the pacing electrode is attached to extension leads and connected to the generator. The pacing energy is always set at least twice the threshold level (the lowest electrical energy needed to pace).

Chest X-ray subsequently confirms the position of the wire.

The care of the patient with a permanent system

This may have been done under general or local anaesthetic. A chest X-ray, usually in the X-ray department, and an electrocardiograph will be performed on return to the ward. Vital signs, BP, pulse and wound are checked half-hourly for four hours then less frequently. Analgesia will be dispensed as necessary. Sometimes a Redivac drain is inserted during the operation; this is removed within 24 hours.

Before discharge, a pacemaker check is done. The patient will receive a booklet and also a card with his pacemaker make and number. He should be instructed to carry this with him at all times. Some patients carry an identity bracelet. He should also be aware that some electronic devices may interfere with his pacemaker, for example in public libraries or some airports. The patient should not drive until the first pacemaker check is performed at one month. The POD pacemaker dressing is removed, the wound sprayed with nobecutane skin protection. Steri-strips are usually *in situ*, to be removed at approximately 5–7 days by the district nurse or general practitioner (no sutures to be removed). Sutures can be removed at 7 days (if surgeons do not use absorbable subcuticular sutures).

Coronary angioplasty (PTCA)

Angioplasty is the technique of dilating blocked or narrow arteries by a balloon catheter which is inflated within the narrowing. It should be carried out in centres where cardiac catheterisation is performed on a regular basis and where a surgical team is available if necessary.

For elective PTCA the patient is given soluble aspirin 300 mg daily if not contraindicated.

The nursing rôle can be divided into:

1. The preparation of the patient for angiography and angioplasty (done separately or as a continuous procedure).
2. The care of the patient after angiography and/or angioplasty.

Preparation before angiography/angioplasty

A full explanation of the procedure(s) should be given to both patient and the relative. A consent form for PTCA and possible CABG should be signed. The patient should be fasted and comprehensively shaved (either a brachial or femoral route will be used). In the case of unstable angina this will be from neck to ankles, in case surgery is required. Take MSU, nose and throat swabs, height, weight, ECG, X-ray, haemoglobin, U and E and blood group.

The 'stand-by' surgeon and anaesthetist will visit the patient. An intravenous cannula will be inserted and the nurse should ensure its patency, sterility and accuracy of infusion rate. The patient's foot pulses will be checked and marked for future reference.

Premedication and the theatre check-list are done by two nurses and an identification bracelet is affixed.

Post-angiography/angioplasty

Special instructions may be directed on the operation form, and should be sought.

Vital signs
Initially the blood pressure, apex rate and peripheral warmth and colour and pedal pulses will be recorded half-hourly. The frequency of this will become less if the patient remains stable and will then be every four hours. A cardiac monitor is observed and changes reported to the doctor. (Elective angioplasty patients are usually beta-blocked – HR 50–60 b.p.m., sinus bradycardia.)

The wound site should be observed half-hourly initially, then less frequently, for bleeding or haematoma. Sometimes the sheath is left inserted in case of further intervention. If bleeding does occur, pressure and a firm pressure bandage should be applied. If no problem arises then the bandage can be removed 12–24 hours later. When a sheath is removed the patient must lie flat for a further four hours with half-hourly BP, apex, foot pulse and wound checks.

The patient usually receives intravenous:

1. Heparin during procedure.
2. Dextrose 70 (1000 ml for 6 hours).
3. Isoket infusion for up to 24 hours post-PTCA and sometimes heparin.

Chest pain
A 12-lead electrocardiograph should be recorded on return to the unit. If further chest pain does occur a further ECG, with any

changes, should be reported to the medical staff. Isoket may need to be increased. Another ECG is routinely taken after 24 hours.

Mobility
The patient should be nursed flat immediately after angioplasty for four hours, then gradually elevated with pillows, with care similar to that of any patient on bed rest, and he can sit out of bed the following day.

Eating and drinking
If the angioplasty result is not as good as expected, or problems occurred during the procedure, the patient may have to be kept starved for four hours; otherwise he/she may eat or drink. If not thin, the patient should be given a Marriott diet before discharge.

The patient's stay in hospital is short, usually 3–4 days. The nurse should ensure all adequate preparation and indoctrination is made before discharge. Booklets and diet cards are now available for patient reference.

Myocardial infarction

The aim of the nursing team is to alleviate pain, to detect arrhythmias, to observe the complications and to rehabilitate the patient so that he can return to as normal a life-style as possible.

Blood pressure, temperature and respiration are recorded on admission; these not only act as a baseline for planning care but act as parameters for any change in clinical status. Urine and blood glucose and electrolyte levels are measured.

Observations

The patient should be made as comfortable as possible and attached to a cardiac monitor for detection of arrhythmias. A 12-lead ECG should be recorded immediately; this will not only confirm the diagnosis but, with the history, may indicate whether thrombolytic therapy would reduce the size of the infarction.

Prompt detection of arrhythmias in the early stages of infarction is essential since they are life threatening. Any arrhythmia, early or late, should be documented by rhythm strip, reported to the medical staff and its treatment instigated as necessary.

Therapy

Proper fluid balance sheets should be filled hourly or half-hourly. An intravenous route must be established quickly for the administration of drugs and fluids.

Reassurance is of paramount importance at all times: the patient may be frightened of dying, even if these fears are not voiced; he should be told that he has had a heart attack but emphasis is placed on his return home and to a normal life-style.

Pain is the major presenting symptom in the majority of patients with myocardial infarction. It should be dealt with efficiently, not only for humanitarian reasons but because releases of catecholamines may lead to arrhythmias and extension of the muscle necrosis. No one can experience the pain of another and for this reason every pain is different and may be heightened by fear. Intravenous diamorphine has been found to be the most effective practice.

In non-complicated myocardial infarction, bed rest is recommended for the first 24 hours following admission to the ITU. During this period the physiotherapists will have encouraged deep breathing exercises, as well as passive limb movements to combat complications of bed rest, including deep vein thrombosis.

Recovery

The second day will normally see the patient sitting out of bed and, on transfer to the progressive ward, he will continue his mobilisation under the supervision of the nurse and the physiotherapist.

During the early stages of infarction the patient will be offered daily bed-baths and washes. Although the nurse realises the importance of hygiene, sometimes the patient is too exhausted or under the influence of drugs, so he should be left to rest until he feels able to participate. Once the patient is mobile, he can be involved in his own care, and should be asked about the other problems he may have with his health.

Many units now encourage the use of commodes rather than bedpans, as their use is considered less strenuous. Aperients should be available to combat constipation early after infarction.

At this time many patients do not want to eat and may feel nauseated; this can be overcome by the use of an anti-emetic. Once the patient is over the acute stage of infarction dietary advice can be given, including reducing, low fat and high fibre diets.

Patients who stop smoking have a lower mortality than those

who continue. Advice is essential and can be given in a discussion group or on an individual basis, and/or with booklets. Advice will include work, leisure, diet, exercise and smoking, all of which can lead to confidence about the future. Health education and rehabilitation is one of the most important rôles we can undertake to help the patient return to his place in society. If the help of other health care workers is required, for example the social worker, this should be obtained as soon after admission as possible.

Before discharge it is advisable to see both patient and relatives together and, if possible, invite them to a group discussion as this prevents misunderstanding of information given.

Cardiac surgery

Abbreviations in cardiac medicine

IVC	Inferior vena cava
SVC	Superior vena cava
RA	Right atrium
TV	Tricuspid valve
RV	Right ventricle
PV	Pulmonary valve
PA	Pulmonary artery
RPA	Right pulmonary artery
LPA	Left pulmonary artery
LA	Left atrium
MV	Mitral valve
LV	Left ventricle
Ao	Aorta
RVOT	Right ventricular outflow tract
LVOT	Left ventricular outflow tract
SVR	Systemic vascular resistance
EF	Ejection fraction
SV	Stroke volume; systolic volume
SI	Stroke index; systolic index
SW	Stroke work
CVP	Central venous pressure
HR	Heart rate
P	Pulse rate
RAP	Right atrial pressure
RVP	Right ventricular pressure
RVEDP	Right ventricular end-diastolic pressure
PASP	Pulmonary artery systolic pressure
PADP	Pulmonary artery diastolic pressure
PAWP	Pulmonary artery wedge pressure
PVR	Pulmonary vascular resistance
LAP	Left atrial pressure
LVEDP	Left ventricular end-diastolic pressure

AoV   Aortic volume
CO   Cardiac output
CI   Cardiac index
BP   Blood pressure
MAP   Mean arterial pressure
LVSW Left ventricular systolic work
RVSW Right ventricular systolic work

See also section on Cardiorespiratory formulae.

Tables of normal values

Table 2.1 Normal cardiovascular pressures (mmHg)

PA	
Systolic	25 (15–30)
Diastolic	10 (5–15)
Mean	15 (10–20)
Wedge	10 (5–15)
LA	7 (4–12)
LV	
Systolic	120 (90–140)
End–diastolic	7 (4–12)
RA	4 (0–8)
RV	
Systolic	25 (15–30)
End–diastolic	4 (0–8)
Aorta	
Systolic	120 (90–140)
Diastolic	70 (60–90)
Mean	85 (70–105)
Blood pressure	
Systolic	(90–140)
Diastolic	(60–90)

Table 2.2 Left ventricular volumes

End-diastolic volume (LVEDP)	70–85 ml/m^2
End-systolic volume (LVESV)	25–30 ml/m^2
Systolic volume (LVSV)	45–55 ml/m^2
Ejection fraction (EF)	0.65–0.75
Stroke work (LVSW)	50–80 g/m/m^2
Effective stroke volume	45–55 ml/m^2
Regurgitant volume	Nil

Table 2.3 Distribution of cardiac output

Organ	Weight (kg)	Body weight (%)	Blood flow (ml/min)	Cardiac output (%)
Brain	1.4	2	775	15.0
Heart	0.3	0.43	175	3.3
Kidneys	0.3	0.43	1100	23.0
Liver	1.5	2.1	1400	29.0
Lungs	1.0	1.5	175	3.3
Muscles	27.8	39.7	1000	19.0
Rest	38.7	55.34	375	9.7

Table 2.4 Normal heart rate according to age

Age	Heart rate (beats/min)
<1 month	120–190
1–6 months	110–180
6 months–1 year	100–170
1–3 years	90–160
3–6 years	80–150
6–15 years	70–140

Table 2.5 Average blood pressure (not necessarily 'ideal') according to age

Age	Blood pressure (mmHg)	MAP
Less than 6 months	80/46	57
6 months to 1 year	89/60	70
1 to 2 years	99/64	76
2 to 4 years	100/64	77
4 to 12 years	105/65	78
12 to 15 years	118/68	85
More than 15 years	120/70	87

Cardiovascular formulae

MAP (Mean arterial pressure)

$$= DP + \frac{SP - Dp}{3}$$

Normal: 80–90 mmHg

CO (Cardiac output)

= Stroke volume × Heart rate

Fick method:

$$= \frac{O_2 \text{ consumption (ml/min)}}{(AV) O_2 \text{ content (ml/litre)}} = \frac{Vo_2}{Cao_2 - Cvo_2}$$

Normal: 4–7 litres/min

CI (Cardiac index)

$$= \frac{CO}{BSA}$$

Normal: 2.5–4.0 litres/m^2

VR (Vascular resistance in general)

$$= \frac{\text{Pressure}}{\text{Flow}}$$

SVR (Systemic vascular resistance)

$$= \frac{MAP - CVP}{CO} \times 80$$

Normal: 1000–2000 dyne/cm^{-5}

PVR (Pulmonary vascular resistance)

$$= \frac{PAP - LAP}{CO} \times 80$$

Normal: 155–255 dyne/cm^{-5}

PCWP (Pulmonary capillary wedge pressure)
Measured by flotation catheter
Normal: 5–15 mmHg

PCP (Pulmonary capillary pressure)
= PCWP + 0.4 (PAP − PCWP)
Normal: 8–18 mmHg

SV (Stroke volume)
= LVEDV − LVESV
Normal: 50–60 ml

SI (Stroke index)

$$= \frac{SV}{BSA}$$

Normal: 35–40 ml/m^2

SW (Stroke work)
= SV × MAP
Normal: 400–500 units

LVSW (Left ventricular stroke work)
= SV × (MAP − PCWP) × 0.136
Normal: 50–80 units

LVSW (from CO values)

$$= \frac{CO \times MAP \times 0.136}{HR}$$

RVSW (Right ventricular stroke work)

$$= \frac{CO \times MAP \times 0.136}{HR}$$

Normal: 5–15 units

LVSWI (Left ventricular stroke work index)

$$= \frac{LVSW}{BSA}$$

Normal: 30–40

EF (Ejection fraction)

$$= \frac{LVEDV - LVESV}{LVEDV} \times 100$$

Normal: 65–75%

Oxygen delivery

$$= Cao_2 \times CO \times 10$$

Normal: 1000 ml/min

D (a–v) o_2 (Arteriovenous oxygen difference)

$$= (1.34 \times Hb) \times (Sao_2 - Svo_2)$$

Normal: 3.5–4.5 ml/100 ml

Vo_2 (Oxygen consumption)

$$= D \text{ (a–v) } o_2 \times CO \times 10$$

Normal: 250 ml/min

Oxygen utilization

$$= \frac{D \text{ (a–v) } o_2}{Cao_2 \times CO}$$

Normal: Below 0.3

Cao_2 (Arterial oxygen content)

$$= (Pao_2 \times 0.0031) + (Hb \times 1.34 \times \% \text{ art. sat.})$$

Cvo$_2$ (Venous oxygen content)

= $(P$vo$_2 \times 0.0031) + ($Hb $\times 1.34 \times \%$ ven. sat.$)$

Cco$_2$ (Alveolar blood oxygen content)

= $(P$ao$_2 \times 0.0031) + ($Hb $\times 1.34 \times 100)$

Mixed venous oxygen content

= Cao$_2 - \dfrac{V$o$_2}{\text{CO}}$

Qs/Qt (Physiological shunt)

= $\dfrac{Cc - Ca}{Cc - Cv} \times 100$

Qp/Qs (Pulmonary to systemic flow ratio)

= $\dfrac{\text{Systemic artery } So_2 - \text{RA } So_2}{\text{LA } So_2 - \text{PA } So_2}$

Pao$_2$ (Oxygen alveolar pressure)

= $[(\text{Bar press} - P$H$_2$o$) \times F$io$_2] - P$aco$_2$

(A–a)Do$_2$ (Alveolo-arterial oxygen gradient)

= Pao$_2 - P$ao$_2$

Qs/Qt from respiratory values

= $\dfrac{\text{Unoxygenated cardiac output}}{\text{Total cardiac output}}$

= $\dfrac{\text{(A–a) } \text{do}_2 \times 0.0031}{[\text{(A–a) } \text{do}_2 \times 0.0031] + (Cao_2 - Cvo_2)}$

= $\dfrac{(P$ao$_2 - P$ao$_2) \times 0.0031}{[(P$ao$_2 - P$ao$_2) \times 0.0031] + (C$ao$_2 - C$vo$_2)}$

Cardiopulmonary bypass

Open heart surgery has become possible thanks to a series of achievements occurring since Le Gallois proposed in 1812 that, with an adequate pump, it would be a reality in the future. The development of oxygenators, the discovery of heparin and the first experiments in animals have led to the sophisticated procedures nowadays performed round the world.

The basic principle

Bypassing the heart by draining the blood from the venae cavae, oxygenating it in the machine and retransfusing through the aorta is usually carried out via routine median sternotomy with the blood heparinised (3 mg/kg to keep the activated clotting time around 450 s).

The arterial line is usually inserted in the aortic root, though in emergency cases the femoral artery may be cannulated. The venous drainage is accomplished via the right atrium, either cannulating the inferior and superior venae cavae individually, or simply draining the right atrial blood through a single pipe. In cases of crashing emergencies, especially in massive bleeding from the chest during opening for reoperations, the femoral vein serves for partial bypass. Once the aorta is cross-clamped, the cardioplegic solution is given through the aortic root and the heart is decompressed by the apex (valve surgery), right superior pulmonary vein (valve surgery), right atrium (most open heart operations), left atrium (cardiac transplantation), or pulmonary artery.

The cannulation itself might create problems: arterial dissection, air embolism, bleeding.

Adequate rate, pressure and content of perfusate is vital during the procedure. The perfusionist controls blood volume, systemic blood flow, arterial tone, venous tone, arterial blood pressure, venous blood pressure, pulsatility, blood viscosity, haematocrit and temperature.

The haematocrit is maintained at 25% to compensate for the increased viscosity and vasoconstriction caused by the hypothermia. The perfusion pressure should be kept at 50–60 mmHg and never below 30 mmHg, since this can be deleterious for the brain. The pump flow rate is kept at 2.4 litres/min/m^2 and the systemic temperature between 20°C and 28°C.

The oxygenators used in the pump may be: direct gas interface type (rotating disc, screen and bubble), in which the blood is in direct contact with the gases in the machine; and membrane type, in which there is an interface between the gases and the blood.

One of the most important components of bypass is hypothermia. The time of ischaemic tolerance of tissues at normothermia (5 minutes for the brain) is doubled for each 5°C of cooling. Thus the brain is protected for 6–9 min at 32°C and 40 min at 23°C.

Total circulatory arrest is used in many congenital malformations to avoid blood shunting and in aortic aneurysms. Brief cardiac arrest without hypothermia is an unavoidable manoeuvre in extreme emergencies (atrial and ventricular tears, massive bleeding during pneumonectomy, 'crash' pulmonary embolectomy).

After the intracardiac operation and when haemostasis seems adequate, the patient is weaned off bypass and the cardiac performance observed. Any complications will be treated accordingly, e.g. pacing wires for heart block, inotropics for low cardiac output, etc. The heart is eventually decannulated, haemostasis perfected and the patient closed, leaving at least two drains, one in the mediastinum and another one at the back of the heart.

Myocardial protection during open heart surgery

The basal coronary flow is 80 ml/min per 100 g of cardiac muscle, which is ten times higher than the rest of the body; 75% of the oxygen is extracted from the blood, so additional requirements are provided from increased coronary flow.

During cardiopulmonary bypass, a low perfusion pressure, ventricular distension or fibrillation, added to poor vasculature in cases of coronary obstruction, increase myocardial vulnerability, particularly to maintain metabolic requirements. This ischaemic damage is reversible during the first 10 to 15 minutes. After 60 minutes the cellular glycogen virtually disappears, myofibrils degenerate, mitochondria show severe oedema and the cytoplasmic membrane disintegrates.

To complicate matters, if this severely damaged myocardium is suddenly perfused, the oedema worsens, calcium phosphate accumulates and the cells 'explode'. The process can be attenuated by reducing myocardial activity and metabolic requirements and increasing oxygen and substrates during ischaemia.

Rapid inactivation of the myocardium before anaerobiosis preserves high-energy phosphates and glycogen and minimises suprabasal metabolic requirements. Cellular damage is also prevented by buffering both the intracellular and extracellular environment. Hypothermia is one of the most important parts of myocardial and systemic protection; it reduces basal metabolism.

Hypothermia is achieved in three ways: by systemic, epicardial and intramyocardial cooling. With modern cardioplegia the heart is satisfactorily protected for 120 minutes during cardiopulmonary bypass, as long as hypothermia is kept uniform during the procedure. However, when the heart is not completely isolated from warmer areas (mediastinum, diaphragm, tubing from the heart–lung machine), the warming may cause severe metabolic injury and even necrosis. This is prevented by insulating the heart from the pericardium, giving adequate amounts of cardioplegic solutions, isolating caval venous flow and keeping a low systemic flow in order to avoid collateral flow, which may be 400 ml/min and can be reduced 30% by limiting systemic flow to 1.5 litres/m/m^2.

Usually, a systemic temperature of 24°C and a local (myocardial) temperature of 10°C protect the heart safely.

Artificial cardiac arrest may be achieved by many methods:

1. Cardiac ischaemia (intermittent aortic clamping).
2. Deep hypothermia.
3. Direct electric depolarisation.
4. Ventricular fibrillation.
5. Cardioplegic solutions.

Intermittent aortic clamping gives very short time of protection and may cause damage to the aorta and severe myocardial ischaemia. Ventricular fibrillation is still used in many centres but does not have the flexibility of other methods. Continuous coronary perfusion is becoming a method of the past. It might be used for valve surgery. Deep hypothermic arrest is mainly used in paediatric cardiac surgery and in some cases of aortic surgery.

Cardioplegic arrest and protection is the most popular, safe and easy method used nowadays. It can provide substrates, allows a good operating time, keeps the heart immobile and protects the myocardium from ischaemic damage. Cardioplegic solutions may be colloid or crystalloid. The former are best represented by blood cardioplegia. The latter can be divided into those of intracellular and extracellular constituents (see Table 2.6). 'Intracellular' solutions produce cardiac arrest by reducing ionic gradients through cellular membranes, using low sodium and calcium concentrations (e.g. Bretschneider and Kirsch solutions). 'Extracellular' solutions cause arrest by depolarisation due to high potassium and magnesium concentrations (St Thomas').

Whichever solution is used, it is infused through the ascending aorta or directly into the coronaries if the aorta is opened. The

Table 2.6 Substrate concentration of two typical cardioplegic solutions

Substrate	Concentration (mmol/litre)
Bretschneider (intracellular)	
NaCl	15
KCl	8
$MgCl_2$	8
Histidine	180
Tryptophane	2
Mannitol	20
St Thomas' (extracellular)	
Na^+	110
K^+	16
Ca^{2+}	1.2
Mg^{2+}	16
Cl^-	160
$NaHCO_3$	10

usual amount is 1 litre given over 3 to 5 minutes, which creates a pressure of 50 mmHg. It may be reinfused every half-hour, with the additional advantages of maintaining the arrest, keeping the hypothermia level, cleaning the extracellular fluid from acid metabolites, providing substrates, and preserving the osmolarity, preventing cellular oedema. It may be more logical to use an intracellular solution to refresh cardioplegia initiated with an extracellular type.

If the myocardium has not been adequately protected, the reperfusion period is critical: the sudden changes in pressure, flow, oxygenation, osmolarity and substrate concentration can lead to massive enzyme liberation, production of superoxides and free radicals, which may damage the heart irreversibly.

Reperfusion

'Venting' the heart during reperfusion or blood cardioplegia is important, since it prevents distension, which may redistribute the subendocardial flow, causing ischaemia during rewarming. Venting may be achieved through the ventricular apex, right superior pulmonary vein, left atrium, pulmonary artery or ascending aorta.

The cardioplegic solution is usually vented through the superior vena cava cannulation site in the right atrium.

The sudden exposure to calcium after using intracellular solutions may cause the so-called 'calcium paradox', with disruption of the cellular membrane and massive calcium inflow to the cell, impairing the cellular situation even more.

The damage from calcium re-entry, free radicals and superoxides, over-distension, acidosis, oedema, fibrillation, etc., with resultant 'explosive' myocardial disintegration, can be minimised by reperfusion at normothermia, with normal pressures, additional magnesium, slightly alkalotic, slightly hyperosmotic perfusate, containing mannitol as a free-radical sponge, and avoiding distension and fibrillation of the recovering heart.

Postoperative care: overall picture

Basic observations

The basic observations after heart surgery must include:

1. General condition: peripheral circulation, distress, bleeding, conscious level, movements, chest inspection.
2. Drainage rate through mediastinal drains.
3. ECG monitoring: rate, rhythm, QRS/ST patterns, pacing wires connected appropriately.
4. Mean arterial pressure around 75–85 mmHg.
5. Central venous pressure around 10–15 mmHg.
6. Left atrial pressure around 15–23 mmHg.
7. Urine output about 0.5–1.0 ml/kg/h.
8. Fluids and electrolytes: 1.0–2.0 ml/kg/h of iso-osmolar solution. Potassium should be kept between 4.0–4.5 mmol/litre.
9. Ventilations: V_T of 10–15 ml/kg; IMV: 8–12/min.
10. Blood balance.
11. Blood gases.
12. Chest X-rays.
13. Nursing care: pressure points, mucous membranes, etc.
14. Physiotherapy and respiratory therapy.

General care of the cardiovascular system

Fundamental to the maintenance of life is the supply of necessities to every cell in the body. There must be enough blood of the right constitution propelled to every cell at the right speed and at the right temperature. Failure of any of these requirements will soon show by various reflexes and later by evidence of metabolic derangement. Ideally, even the reflex evidence should not be allowed to appear. The reflex manifestations of cell deprivation of anything include the feeling of dyspnoea which may result in 'fighting' the ventilator, vasoconstriction which may itself worsen the cells' supply failure, sweating, reduced urinary output, anxiety and tachycardia (late in infants: bradycardia). The late, metabolic, manifestations include acidosis, hyperkalaemia, falling mixed venous oxygen saturation and arterial saturation and the effects of deprivation on essential organs like the liver, kidneys and brain.

The supply failure involving the composition of the blood most commonly is a deficiency of oxygen. (Supply, carrying power or availability.) Other nutrients include glucose (and a means of making it available, i.e. insulin) and the precursors of metabolic enzymes such as vitamins.

Hypovolaemia

The delivery of the blood is the task of the cardiovascular system. There must be enough blood to fill the vessels and to give the ventricles enough filling pressure to prime them fully. The normal blood volume is 7% of the body weight or 3 litres per square metre. A fall below this would cause reflex vasoconstriction and tachycardia initially, with metabolic changes if more than these mechanisms could compensate for. When more than 10% of the intravascular volume is lost, the clinical manifestations of hypovolaemia are present. The hypovolaemic patient is hypotensive, hypoperfused, tachycardic, with collapsed neck veins, weak pulses and small urine output.

The most important causes of hypovolaemia in the cardiac postoperative patient are:

1. *Bleeding.* As stated earlier, the presence of more than 200 ml per hour in the thoracic drains for four consecutive hours, or more than 400 ml at any time, generally demands reopening. Sometimes the cause of bleeding is in one of the multiple holes the surgeon has to make (aortic cannulation, aortic cardioplegia, atrial cannulation, cardiotomies, ventricular or pulmonary artery vents, coronary anastomosis, etc). On the other hand, defective clotting factors may be responsible. The adequacy of heparin reversal affects the accelerated clotting time (ACT), which can be cellite or saline. Abnormalities of the coagulation tests should be corrected by administration of specific factors (e.g. protamine, platelets, fresh frozen plasma or whole blood).
2. *Other causes.* Particularly water loss and/or excessive vasodilatation. The choice of volume for replacement depends on the cause and the packed cell volume (PCV). Blood or plasma expanders should be used to arrive at a PCV around 35%.

Hypervolaemia

The other extreme of the spectrum is hypervolaemia. A rise above the normal limits can easily cause congestive cardiac failure, with oedema of whichever part of the body is congested (usually the lungs first, as the left heart normally fails first). The pressure in the veins and left atrium are guides to the adequacy of the blood volume and normally parallel each other, but sometimes the right or left heart fails alone and, if the latter, filling a patient up until he has a normal right heart filling pressure may elevate the left filling pressure to the level producing pulmonary oedema. In these uncommon situations, therefore, a left atrial pressure is invaluable but technically difficult to obtain unless a tube has been left at operation. However, Swan–Ganz catheterisation provides pulmonary wedge pressure; or the pulmonary artery end-diastolic pressure from a floated-in catheter can be used, except in pulmonary hypertension (in which circumstances the right-sided filling pressure would be the critical one anyway).

Once a good output and normally filled peripheral veins demonstrate normovolaemia, the filling pressures may be allowed to fall to levels which reflect the excellence of the heart. The maximum permissible filling pressures depend somewhat on the integrity of the semipermeability of the capillaries in that, after a poor perfusion, oedema may develop in tissues at much lower capillary pressures than normally. The same will be seen if the plasma colloid osmotic pressure is reduced by hypoalbuminaemia. Normally, however, right-sided pressures of 15 mmHg and left-sided ones of 24 mmHg should not be exceeded, unless seen in hypovolaemia plus vasoconstriction, when vasodilators will allow appropriate fluids to be given.

Myocardial failure: low cardiac output syndrome

In the presence of a normal volume of normally composed blood, tissue malperfusion is the result of heart failure. This in turn may be due to haemodynamic, arrhythmic or myocardial disorder and the myocardium may be afflicted by cellular damage or vascular insufficiency. The distinction is usually obvious clinically and if a remediable 'plumbing' problem underlies the heart failure, no time should be lost in correcting it surgically, especially if its remedy is simple, as in the case of postoperative tamponade from blood.

An *arrhythmic* problem is usually immediately apparent and capable of solution. Post-operative *non-ischaemic myocardial insufficiency* is the most common and least welcome of all the causes of postoperative cardiac failure. It may be the result of prolonged operative ischaemia with inadequate myocardial protection, air in the coronary vessels, damage to coronaries by cannulae, part of a generalised body insult from prolonged cardiopulmonary bypass ('total body confusion') with pump–oxygenator systems of high damage potential rather than newer disposable clear-fluid prime membrane or bubble oxygenators and accurate roller, pulsatile or centrifugal pumps. It is characterised by low fixed stroke volume, low diastolic compliance and slow contraction velocity (a stiff ventricle). Although inotropic agents may speed up and strengthen myocardial contraction, they may make an already spastic ventricle even more so, especially if it is already hypertrophic as in severe aortic stenosis, when the large muscle mass relative to coronary supply may complete the prerequisites for subendocardial necrosis. As high a filling pressure as the capillary permeability will stand (pulmonary oedema shows promptly by increased alveolar–arterial Po_2 gradient) and a peripheral dilator like glyceryl trinitrate or sodium nitroprusside to reduce ventricular workload are at least as important as catecholamines in the management of this problem. Correction of acidosis, hyperkalaemia, arrhythmias and anoxia are essential preliminary measures. If all these moves fail, balloon counterpulsation will augment cardiac output considerably, and a left ventricular assist device can be used if the situation seems reversible.

Ischaemic myocardial insufficiency is not seen often after open heart operations but is a common sight in coronary care units. Management is the same as for the non-ischaemic variety but glucose–insulin–potassium may have a place, with anti-arrhythmics, of higher importance. The fundamental cause of the problem – blocked coronary arteries – may be a surgical problem, even at this late stage, if a large amount of ischaemia surrounds the infarction, the coronary blocks during coronary angiography or angioplasty on the threshold of theatre, or initial success with thrombolysis is failing.

Haemodynamic causes of postoperative cardiac failure include tamponade, which shows by falling output, rising pulse and venous pressures, excessive 'pulsus paradoxus', Kussmaul venous sign, and a marked fall in pressures with isoprenaline rather than the improvement seen when myocardial failure underlies the low output.

Reopening in ITU

Postoperative cardiac tamponade is notoriously difficult to identify, though will never be found if not thought of. Even ultrasound is not a completely reliable way of excluding this problem and reopening may be the only way to do so. Bleeding of over 200 ml per hour, not diminishing or increasing, is an indication for reopening, but in this context and in that of deliberately exploring for tamponade, the facilities of the theatre should be used.

Before deciding to reopen a patient for bleeding, remember what in our unit are called the 'multiple Ps': plasma, protamine, platelets, precipitate (cryo) and PEEP.

(Some of our registrars have continued the list with: procedure, pressure, prolene, patches and prayers.)

Massive bleeding, or the deterioration of the heart to a lethal degree without adequate explanation, justifies reopening of the sternotomy in ITU. Experience has shown that this resource has not resulted in more wound infection provided the usual standards of asepsis normal in theatre are applied in the unit. Sterile thoracotomy packs are available and proper scrub and gown measures can usually be followed. It is important for those planning equipment to ensure that the packs include wire cutters for sternotomy wires and that the suction available is strong enough to evacuate big clots.

Table 2.7 Effects of inotropes used in intensive care

	Adrenaline	Noradrenaline	Isoprenaline	Dopamine	Dobutamine	Salbutamol
Vaso-constriction	+++	++++	0	0 to +++	+	0
Vasodilation	+	0	++++	++	+	++++
Renal dilatation	0	0	0	++++	0	0
Rate increase	++++	++++	++++	++++	++++	0
Contractility	++++	++++	++++	++++	++++	0
Arrhythmias	++++	++++	++++	++	+	+
Preload	Variable	Increased	Decreased	Variable	Variable	Variable
Afterload	Variable	Increased	Decreased	Variable	Variable	Variable

Note: Alpha effect is vasoconstriction; beta-2 effect is vasodilatation; beta-1 effect is heart contractility, rate and conduction; delta effect is renal vasodilatation.

Formulae

1. For adrenaline, noradrenaline and isoprenaline:
   (BW in kg × 3)/100 = mg to add to 50 ml of solution
   >   Then: 1 ml/h = 0.01 µm/kg/min
   >   Range: 2–20 ml/h
2. For dopamine and dobutamine:
   (BW in kg × 3) = mg to add to 50 ml solution
   >   Then: 1 ml/h = 1 µm/kg/min
   >   Range: 2–20 ml/h

Table 2.8 Doses of main inotropes

	Dose (µg/kg/min)	Dose (µg/h)	Dilution	Speed range (ml/h)
Adrenaline	0.02–0.2	72–1280	1 mg/100 ml (10 µg/ml)	7–120
Noradrenaline	0.01–0.2	36–1280	1 mg/100 ml (10 µg/ml)	4–120
Isoprenaline	0.02–0.2	72–1280	1 mg/100 ml (10 µg/ml)	7–120
Dopamine	2–20	7–128 (mg/h)	200 mg/100 ml (2 mg/ml)	3–60
Dobutamine	2–20	7–128 (mg/h)	250 mg/100 ml (2.5 mg/ml)	3–50
Salbutamol	0.02–0.2	72–1280	1 mg/100 ml (10 µg/ml)	7–120

Note: If it is necessary to restrict the amount of fluids then double the doses or halve the diluent.

Table 2.9 Speed range (ml/h) when drug strength changes

	1 mg/100 ml	2 mg/100 ml	4 mg/100 ml	8 mg/100
Adrenaline Noradrenaline Isoprenaline Salbutamol	7–120	3–60	2–30	1–15

Vasodilators used in postoperative cardiac surgery

Formula for sodium nitroprusside

(BW in kg × 3)/10 = mg to add to 50 ml of solution
>   Then: 1 ml/h = 0.1 µg/kg/min
>   Range: 1–15 ml/h

Table 2.10 Vasodilators used in postoperative cardiac surgery

	Artery	Vein	Onset (min)	Duration	Dose
Nitroprusside	+	+	1	2–5 min	0.3–15.0 µg/kg/min
Nitroglycerine	–	+	1–2	10 min	0.3–4.0 µg/kg/min
Diazoxide	+	–	1	4–12 h	300 mg i.v. up to 3 times
Trimetaphan	+	–	1	2–5 min	1–15 mg/min
Hydralazine	+	–	10–20	2–6 h	5–20 mg i.v.
Phentolamine	+	–	1–2	20 min	0.1–2.0 mg/min up to 60 mg

The intra-aortic balloon pump

The general principle of the intra-aortic balloon pump (IABP) is to evacuate the stroke volume from the aorta in systole, thus making room for the effortless ejection of that volume by the ventricle, and then in diastole to replace this volume in the aorta after aortic valve closure, thus doing work against pressure and boosting diastolic pressure with particular benefit to the predominantly diastolic coronary flow.

Access to the arterial system is obtained with the smallest possible 'invasion' by a thin catheter with a 50 ml balloon at its terminal 10 cm. The balloon is located in the descending aorta from the subclavian down to the supradiaphragmatic aorta. A low density, low viscosity gas like helium permits more rapid and complete balloon excursions, but carbon dioxide is less risky if the balloon leaks. The balloon excursions are monitored either by having an external 'master' balloon connected to the working 'slave' balloon, or by means of monitoring systems within the drive unit. The drive unit is triggered by the QRS complex of the ECG and the clinician can set the delay between this and the deflation of the balloon, the duration of the deflation and the subsequent reflation.

The ideal is obviously for the balloon to deflate as ventricular systole generates pressure equal to the aortic pressure and to reflate at the moment the aortic valve closes. In practice, the arterial trace is watched and the balloon timing moved to achieve a maximal diastolic 'balloon wave'.

Cardiac energy is spared, the coronary blood flow is increased and systemic perfusion improves from decreased myocardial oxygen consumption, increased cardiac output and reduced pulmonary congestion, diminishing left-to-right shunts and improving aerobic metabolism.

General indications for the IABP are:

- cardiogenic shock secondary to myocardial infarction
- unstable angina with deteriorating condition
- intractable arrhythmias in coronary patients
- acute ventricular septal rupture
- acute mitral valve incompetence
- septic shock
- haemodynamically unstable general surgical patients
- post-cardiopulmonary bypass heart failure
- intraoperative myocardial infarction
- any case of severe low cardiac output.

From the point of view of numbers:

- cardiac index below 1.8 ml/min/m^2
- ejection fraction less than 20%
- LVEDP above 20 mmHg.

Some contraindications for its use are:

- aortic valve incompetence
- dissecting aortic aneurysm
- relatively advanced peripheral vascular disease.

Some reported complications are:

- aortic dissection
- embolism of atheromatous material
- femoral artery obstruction
- infection
- haemorrhage.

Heparin is used while the balloon is in at 30 units/kg loading dose, and at 500–1000 units 2-hourly to keep cellite ACT between 150 and 200.

The respiratory system in cardiac surgery

The lungs of the average cardiac surgical patient are rarely normal, having been exposed to congestive heart failure, high flow rates from left to right shunts, the development of large bronchial collaterals in cyanotic conditions, and even to tobacco-induced bronchitis in the coronary patients. Not only may the pulmonary vascular resistance be raised, but also the airway resistance, from bronchial venous congestion or smoke inhalation.

Operation – especially long bypass with non-autologous blood primes and imperfect management of pumping – increases the lung water content and introduces diffusion defects, and manipulation of the lung at surgery, trauma to the airways, irritation with inhalation anaesthesia, retained secretions and areas of atelectasis resulting from ineffective coughing from pain or sedation combined with totally absorbed inhaled gases all make their contribution to a mixed respiratory insufficiency.

Available data for respiratory evaluation consist of the appearance and respiratory activity of the patient, his blood gas levels, the content and pressure of the inhaled gases and the volume exhaled by the patient, which could be analysed for content though not done at present routinely. The inhaled gases can be varied widely in fully sedated patients on respirators and the consequences observed. In patients ventilating spontaneously the arterial Po_2 relative to the inhaled Po_2 is a guide to the existence of diffusion abnormalities or the presence of shunting in the lung, and the Po_2 is a guide to ventilation–perfusion defects, but artificial ventilation sometimes obscures the latter correlations.

The response of the alveolar–arterial gradient to a brisk diuresis is a way of distinguishing shunting (no response) from alveolar oedema with diffusion defect (improvement) and conversely the response of the gradient to physiotherapy or bag-squeezing is favourable in the atelectatic shunting cases.

Artificial ventilation is frequently applied after open heart operations for the first postoperative night to allow the cardiovascular status to steady up, and as a part of the 'maximum care' philosophy. Its use is indicated for failure of respiratory drive, the inadequacy of ventilatory strength, and intubation at least is required for failure of coughing and when a positive pressure must be applied to the airways in the absence of an oral or nasal means of achieving this. All ventilation techniques are designed to increase lung volumes and minimise intrapulmonary shunt.

The means of delivery of ventilation is now a tube of non-irritating material passed through the nose or (less satisfactory) the mouth; tracheostomy is more likely to be associated with mediastinal infection and is no longer necessary for the prevention of vocal cord abrasion since the modern tubes are well tolerated for many days.

The ventilator should be matched to the patient's requirements. Patients with low or changing pulmonary compliance should have a volume-cycled respirator which will ventilate the same amount regardless of the pressures it generates to achieve it; where there is a leak in the airway, which may be intentional as a loose leaky tube does less damage, especially in babies, then a pressure-cycled respirator is best; when a patient needs help rather than complete control of ventilation, a ventilator which he can trigger is best since the respiratory reflexes are more ideal than the regulation of a machine according to a lot of delayed and fallible blood estimations.

The expired gas should be monitored in all cases with an 'alarm' monitor. After operation in babies, spontaneous ventilation with constant positive airways pressure (CPAP) is better than artificial ventilation. Patients with pulmonary oedema are helped by maintaining a positive end-expiratory pressure (PEEP) with positive pressure ventilation.

Safe weaning from ventilation may be done by leaving the patient to breathe spontaneously (with or without CPAP) but also apply an ever-diminishing baseline of mandatory intermittent ventilation (IMV) to keep him from fatal underventilation.

At all times, when the normal nasal humidification channels are bypassed, the inhaled gases should be fully humidified. All ventilation apparatus should be fully sterilised between uses and aseptic techniques should be used for all intra-airway procedures. Wherever there is total dependence on a ventilator, full alarm systems should exist for the supply of gases, heat and humidification of inspired gases and the volume of expired gas (see also Table 4.2).

Once committed to ventilation, the habitual reluctance to give large doses of analgesics for fear of lowering ventilatory drive need apply no longer, and truly analgesic concentrations can be achieved, with benefit to the tolerance of the tube and ventilator as well as peripheral circulation and general well-being. Though the poppy derivatives are so good, additional cooperation can be wrought from the patient with sedatives like diazepam, and only in the rare circumstance (when it is highly likely that there is something seriously wrong, like blood loss or tamponade) has one to resort to curarising the respirator 'victim' (when it is preferable to use vecuronium rather than curare as the latter may cause peripheral vascular collapse and abdominal distension).

Excessive levels of oxygen may harm the lung and the proportion of oxygen in the inspired air should not exceed that necessary to achieve a Pao_2 of 100–120 mmHg (12–15 kPa).

Far-reaching biochemical disturbances result from over-ventilation to the point of lowering the $Paco_2$, and a slightly higher than normal $Paco_2$ is tolerated by a well-sedated patient and is safer and even beneficial in terms of increased peripheral perfusion and cardiac output. If a large tidal volume as well as high inspired Po_2 is necessary to maintain a satisfactory Pao_2, with the possible consequence of lowering the $Paco_2$, a piece of tube can be added to the connection to the airway tube to increase the dead space.

After correction of large left-to-right shunts the lungs may continue to be oedematous and non-compliant for some time and require both increased airway pressures to relieve oedema and mechanical assistance to move the stiff lungs. Previously oligaemic lungs may become oedematous when full circulation is restored, especially if arterial collaterals from the aorta have not been tied off at the time of corrective operation. Pulmonary hypertension of an active type may reduce pulmonary perfusion relative to ventilation, reduces cardiac output due to right heart inadequacy and also is frequently associated with excessive secretions.

Paediatric surgery

Unless mechanical assistance to shift the air is required, the best support to postoperative children is provided by CPAP, next best is spontaneous ventilation, then artificial ventilation with PEEP and, worst of all, artificial ventilation without PEEP, as judged by low cardiac output and blood gas levels.

The best intubation technique in babies is the Jackson–Rees nasal tube and it is wise to have a fit in the trachea that is not too snug, so that damage to the subglottic area is minimised; when the airways pressure is also above atmospheric, secretions from the throat will not get past the tumour as the air is blowing away. Allowance should be made for the leak when calculating tidal volume required from the paediatric ventilators. Full humidification is essential in children to prevent blockage of the tube.
Some normal volumes in children are:

- Tidal volume: 7 ml/kg (neonates: 6 ml/kg)
- Dead space: tidal volume × 0.3
- Respiratory rate: neonate 30/min; 1–13 years: 24 − (age/2)/min
- Blood volume: 80 ml/kg (neonate: 100 ml/kg).

Calculation of the ventilation volumes should take into account the tubing of the ventilator and the dead space of the system, since the proportion of these relative to the tiny infant is so much more than in larger patients.

With high airway pressures, higher than normal minute volumes may be necessary and dead space may be needed to keep the $Paco_2$ from being reduced.

Discontinuation of ventilation in children may be done with intermittent mandatory ventilation, and continuous airway pressure is a great help. The presence of a small catheter to the bifurcation of the trachea enables a high airway pressure, high oxygen percentage, and repeated suction to be achieved with little interference and should be more often employed, especially in neonates, during weaning from ventilation.

Discontinuation of ventilator

Discontinuing ventilatory assistance may be carried out when the patient looks well, without cardiovascular problem, the airway is clear, respiratory movements uninhibited and Pao_2 is over 300 mmHg (40 kPa) on 100% inspired oxygen. Then a trial of ventilation with a T-tube carrying humidified oxygen–air mixture in the proportion achievable with a face mask (60%) is justified. If then the tidal air is good (over 10 ml/kg), the respiratory rate below 35, the patient not restless, sweating, dyspnoeic or moving his alae nasae, and $Paco_2$ is less than 55 mmHg (7 kPa) and stable, then the tube can be removed. This should be done at the beginning of the working day, when continued evaluation and re-intubation can be done without waiting for off-duty staff.

A reasonable timetable for routine postoperative patients ventilated on the first postoperative night is as follows:

8.00–8.30 a.m. (assuming the patient is awake, cooperative, looks fit and has a clear chest): ventilate with 100% oxygen.

8.30 a.m. blood gas sample, put on to T-tube with 60% oxygen.

9.00 a.m. analyse gases. If the 8.30 Pao_2 is <300 mmHg (40 kPa) the artificial ventilation should be resumed, improve cardiac status or relieve pulmonary oedema, congestion or obstruction. If the 9.00 $Paco_2$ is >55 mmHg (7 kPa), ventilation should be resumed; until the patient is either more wakeful or strong enough to ventilate himself adequately.

Therapeutic bronchoscopy

The accumulation of bronchial secretions may not always be able to be coughed up by the patient or sucked out of the mouth or pharynx by nursing or physiotherapy staff. A sucker can be introduced into the larynx and trachea either under vision or 'blind' and will stimulate coughing and remove the results to good effect. Secretions may be inspissated in the lower bronchial tree, or the patient may be too weak or poorly ventilated to bring even liquid secretions up from there. In these circumstances therapeutic bronchoscopy or 'mini-tracheostomy' has to be done.

In a crashing emergency, which we try to avoid, the patient may be so black that there is no time to spare for anaesthesia, and anyway so far gone that it is not cruel to bronchoscope him without attempting anaesthesia. The ideal is a short general anaesthetic because it is total but without residual depression of movement or sensation, as well as being the most humane.

Local anaesthesia is acceptable in the absence of an anaesthetist. Intravenous valium is supplemented by sucking an anaesthetic lozenge after which a cotton wool soaked in topical lignocaine is held on each pyriform fossa for two minutes, the throat sprayed with topical lignocaine, then the cords sprayed with it using a laryngoscope, and the bronchoscope introduced through which the carina is sprayed and the sucking out proceeded with.

If the procedure has to be done in the patient's bed with the patient conscious, it is best to stand on a stool above the patient's bedhead with the patient sitting up in his usual position. Once the bronchoscope is past the cords the patient is entirely at the mercy of the bronchoscopist and vigilance must be exercised not to be unnecessarily cruel.

Fluids, electrolytes and the renal system in the cardiac surgical patient

Fluid

Balance charts provide much occupational therapy for those producing them but, except in the critical few hours of intensive care, are of little practical value compared with regular scrupulous weighing. Metabolism of food produces up to a pint of water a day and insensible losses may lose this much. The food and the faeces vary in the amount of water contained and patients unconfined vary in their reliability. Fluid intake should be:

- 1 ml/kg/hour in those over 20 kg
- 1.5 ml/kg/hour in those between 10 and 20 kg
- 2 ml/kg/h in those under 10 kg.

Increased initial allowance can be made for moderate dehydration with a dry mouth and bright eyes, which constitutes about 5% of the body weight in children, and severe dehydration with fast pulse, sunken eyes, scant urine and deep respiration, which constitutes about 10% of the weight in children. These deficiencies can be made up in the first 6 hours.

Cardiac patients may have too much water on board, in their extracellular space, where it will do no harm in the periphery; if in the lung, then severe pulmonary dysfunction results and urgent means like reduction of blood volume or afterload or rapid diuresis are required.

If correctly rehydrated and with a normal circulation, 30 ml/h of urine in the adult should be forthcoming and a reduction below this suggests too little water, a poor circulation or some deficiency of renal function.

Electrolytes

Potassium is the most immediately important of these. Most patients with chronic valvular disease who have been on diuretics have a total body deficiency of up to one-third and their tissues soak up the plasma potassium rapidly when a bounding circulation is restored; at the same time much excess water may be eliminated, carrying out more potassium. Thus it is the patients who have experienced the most haemodynamic benefit from surgery who are the most prone to get hypokalaemic and die of ventricular fibrillation. On the other hand, patients with a deteriorating cardiac action get rapidly worse as the resulting cellular acidosis and loss of potassium into the plasma further depress cardiac action.

The urine usually contains about 50 mEq/litre, and this or the measured urinary potassium content should be restored to the patient who is having diuresis, with frequent checks on the plasma level. Replacing urinary losses will also prevent the routine administration of potassium to a patient whose urinary output is falling as his cardiac action deteriorates and his plasma potassium level rises.

Some give 1 mEq of potassium per minute of bypass to patients who have been on diuretics (on the empirical assumption that the longer bypasses need more valves replaced and have probably been on the most diuretics), 10 ml 10% calcium chloride as bypass is ending, and then replace the urinary losses of potassium as they occur (e.g. 5 mEq KCl per 100 ml of urine passed) plus a little to compensate for shift of potassium into cells (e.g. 10 mEq per 50 g of glucose in the postoperative intravenous solution).

Magnesium

This is frequently significantly deficient after open heart surgery, which frequently mimics hypokalaemia, though results in a weaker cardiac contraction and may cause psychological disturbances.

Prevention with 300 mg/day of magnesium chloride orally and up to 35 mg of magnesium as the sulphate per 500 ml of postoperative intravenous fluid, after using 120 mg of magnesium as the sulphate in the heart–lung machine, keeps the postoperative serum levels normal. Great care is necessary to avoid overload when renal function is depressed.

Calcium

There is a large reservoir in everyone's bones, but acute low levels of calcium may depress cardiac function, which is known to depend for contraction on calcium. Therefore, when large volumes of citrated blood are being given it is wise to give 3.5 ml of 10% calcium chloride slowly for each unit of blood used.

Sodium

This is also essential for normal myocardial contraction, sodium is often deficient in patients who have been on diuretics, but caution is advised in heart failure as too much sodium will hold too much water in the patient and may worsen failure. One unit per day of 1/5 normal saline should fill the patient's need for sodium.

Table 2.11 Electrolyte concentrations in fluids

	Extracellular fluid (mmol/litre)	Intracellular fluid (mmol/litre)
Sodium	140	1
Potassium	4	150
Calcium	2	1
Magnesium	1	13
Chloride	101	3
Bicarbonate	27	10
Phosphate	1	50
Sulphate	0.5	10
Organic anions	6	–
Proteins	2	8

As we have already mentioned, it is not uncommon to find electrolyte disturbances after open heart surgery, especially in sodium, potassium, calcium and magnesium. There are clinical signs for recognising them.

1. Hyponatraemia

This may be caused by increased excretion or impaired body regulation. Clinically it presents with tachycardia, increased neuromuscular excitability, headache, abdominal pain, nausea, hypotension, oliguria and shock. It can be classified as:

(a) Hyponatraemia with fluid overloading. In cases of chronic heart or renal failure, overhydration and administration of fluids without electrolytes.

(b) Hyponatraemia with dehydration. In suprarenal failure and extrarenal losses of sodium.

(c) Hyponatraemia with normal hydration. In cases of hyperlipidaemia, hyperproteinaemia and hyperglycaemia.

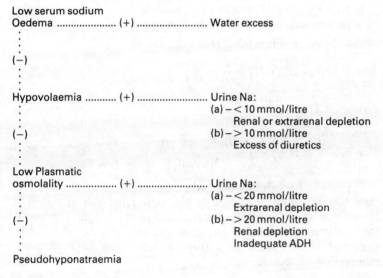

Low serum sodium
Oedema .... (+) .... Water excess

(−)

Hypovolaemia .... (+) .... Urine Na:
(a) − < 10 mmol/litre
Renal or extrarenal depletion
(−)   (b) − > 10 mmol/litre
Excess of diuretics

Low Plasmatic
osmolality .... (+) .... Urine Na:
(a) − < 20 mmol/litre
Extrarenal depletion
(−)   (b) − > 20 mmol/litre
Renal depletion
Inadequate ADH

Pseudohyponatraemia

Figure 2.1

If it is true hyponatraemia, the sodium requirements are:

$$= (\text{Real Na} - 140) \times (\text{BW} \times 0.2)$$

If it is dilutional, the water excess may be calculated by:

$$(\text{BW} \times 0.2) \times \left(1 - \frac{\text{real Na}}{140}\right)$$

and diuretics are given accordingly.

2. Hypernatraemia

This may be real or absolute, or secondary to water loss. Clinically there is intense thirst, central nervous system alterations and hypertonic dehydration at cellular level.

Real hypernatraemia may be due to excessive administration of sodium salts in the presence of impaired renal function, e.g. in Cushing's syndrome, pregnancy and diabetes insipidus, amongst others. Relative hypernatraemia is caused by dehydration, either secondary to fluid loss (increased insensitive losses in patients with mechanical ventilation and fever, osmotic diuresis in diabetics or in patients on total parenteral nutrition) or to poor water ingestion. Treatment varies according to the cause: in real hypernatraemia, sodium ingestion is avoided and natriuretic diuretics are given in order to force renal elimination of sodium.

In hypernatraemia secondary to fluid depletion, some formulae may be applied in order to know the amount of water deficit.

Water deficit (the formulae mean the same):

$$(A) = (0.2 \times BW) \times \left(\frac{Na}{140} - 1 \right)$$

$$(B) = \frac{Na\ real - 140}{140} \times \frac{BW}{5}$$

$$(C) = (0.2 \times BW) - \left(\frac{140 \times 0.2 \times BW}{Na\ real} \right)$$

In cases of hypernatraemia, when the urine osmolality is lower than $800\,mOsm/kg$, the cause is generally renal loss of water. If higher than that, signs of fluid overload must be sought. If present, the patient usually has a real sodium excess; if absent, hypernatraemia is due to extrarenal water loss or inadequate elimination of sodium.

3. Hypokalaemia

This is generally diagnosed through blood measurements in ITU. Nevertheless, there are some clinical signs: weakness, hyporeflexia, muscular hypotonia, dyspnoea, abdominal distension and ECG changes (T wave depression, ST depression, U wave, ventricular ectopics).

In acute cases, potassium is replaced through a central venous line at $20\,mmol/hour$, according to blood levels.

4. Hyperkalaemia (see Renal failure, p. 77)

5. Hypercalcaemia

This shows with anorexia, nausea, vomiting, abdominal pain, intense thirst, polyuria, weakness, neurological alterations, psychotic behaviour, metastatic calcifications and ventricular arrhythmias. Prolonged immobilisation in patients may cause massive movements of calcium into the circulation, particularly if the patient has associated hyperthyroidism, malignancy or hyperparathyroidism.

Treatment is based on adequate hydration with normal saline, forced renal elimination with frusemide and EDTA, dialysis, calcitonin (50–100 units i.m.) and Myntranycin (15–20 µg/litre).

6. Hypocalcaemia

This manifests with tetany, convulsions, mental depression, and the signs of Chvostek and Trousseau. Critical care patients with severe and prolonged alkalosis may suffer hypocalcaemia, particularly if some endocrine conditions such as Cushing's syndrome or hypoparathyroidism are present, and in the presence of chronic renal failure.

Treatment is based on calcium administration, vitamin D, and aluminium hydroxide to block phosphorus absorption.

7. Hypermagnesaemia

This can be seen in renal failure, hypovolaemia and metabolic acidosis. The main signs are nausea, muscular weakness, hyporeflexia, lethargy and coma.

Treatment is based on fluid replacement, correction of acidosis, calcium glutamate, restriction of magnesium ingestion and haemodialysis if necessary.

8. Hypomagnesaemia

This may be caused by acute tubular necrosis, osmotic diuresis, gastrointestinal losses, acute pancreatitis, hepatic cirrhosis, chronic alcoholism, diabetes and hyperthyroidism, amongst many others, including prolonged parenteral nutrition. Clinically there is muscular weakness, abdominal pain, hyperreflexia, tetany, cardiac arrhythmias and alterations of the central nervous system.

Treatment is based on replacement, which can be i.v. in acute situations: 40–80 mmol diluted in 1 litre of 5% dextrose and given over 6 hours.

Renal failure

Less than 30 ml of urine per hour in an adult should arouse suspicion; less than 20 ml per hour is oliguria and less than 10 ml per hour is renal failure, although non-oliguric renal failure may present with rising creatinine and urea. The circulation is confirmed as adequate before impugning the kidneys, and the patient is assumed not to be dehydrated. Escalating doses of frusemide are used, and it is now known that doses up to 1 g can be tolerated. Failure of this response helps to confirm renal failure.

Renal failure following cardiac surgery can be classified as:

(a) Prerenal, generally due to hypoperfusion of the kidney secondary to hypovolaemia or prolonged hypotension following low cardiac output.

(b) Renal, secondary to exacerbation of previous renal disease (nephritis; tubulointerstitial disease; acute tubular necrosis; vascular diseases).

(c) Post-renal, due mainly to obstruction.

The diagnostic study should include:

- urinalysis (specific gravity, proteinuria, casts)
- urea
- serum creatinine
- creatinine clearance
- concentrating ability
- excretion urography
- ultrasound
- isotope renography.

Once diagnosed, *complications* of acute renal failure should be treated first, including:

- infection
- pulmonary oedema
- hypertension
- arrhythmias
- anaemia
- gastrointestinal bleeding
- malnutrition
- neurological complications.

Confirmed renal failure demands the reduction of all fluid to 500 ml a day, with which the day's calories should be given. Excess water can be eliminated by making the patient sweat, so that dialysis can be delayed until the potassium or the urea levels demand it. Some *indications for dialysis* are:

- neurological deficit
- potassium higher than 6.5 mmol/litre
- acidosis with pH < 7.15
- pulmonary oedema
- uraemic pericarditis.

Peritoneal dialysis requires no anticoagulation, is easily managed in the average ITU and provides calories in the glucose absorbed. If the renal failure persists beyond ten days, a renal biopsy should be obtained.

Emergency treatment of hyperkalaemia can be divided thus:

1. Antagonise effects: 20% calcium chloride until ECG changes (max. 60–80 ml).
2. Shift it to cells: – bicarbonate 4.2%, 50–100 ml;
   – insulin/glucose, 20 units in 50 g of glucose decrease potassium by 1 mmol/litre over 1–2 hours.
3. Deplete it: – ion-exchange resins, sodium polystyrine or calcium polystyrine, 50 g in 70% sorbitol or 100 g by enema;
   – dialysis.

Table 2.12 Water and solute concentrations in urine

	Glomerular filtration in 24 h	Amount in 24 h urine	Concentration
Sodium	26 000 mmol	150 mmol	100 mmol/litre
Chloride	18 000 mmol	150 mmol	100 mmol/litre
Bicarbonate	5000 mmol	2 mmol	–
Potassium	720 mmol	120 mmol	70 mmol/litre
Water	180 litres	0.8–1.5 litre	–
Urea	900 mmol	400 mmol	267 mmol/litre
Creatinine	15 μmol	15 μmol	10 μmol/litre
Glucose	900 mmol	–	–
Solutes	50 000 mmol	910 mmol	600 mmol/litre

Formulae

Osmolality

$$= (2 \times Na) + \frac{glucose}{18} + \frac{BUN}{2.8}$$

Sodium excretion fraction

$$= \frac{\text{urine Na (24 h urine vol.)} \times \text{serum creatinine}}{\text{serum Na} \times \text{urine creatinine (24 h urine vol.)}}$$

Creatinine clearance

$$A = \frac{\text{urine creatinine} \times \text{urine vol.}}{\text{serum creatinine}} \times \frac{1.73}{\text{BSA}}$$

$$B = \frac{80 \times (145 - \text{age in years})}{\text{serum creatinine } (\mu\text{mol/litre})}$$

Osmolar clearance

$$= \frac{\text{urine Osm} \times \text{urine vol.} \times 60}{\text{plasma Osm} \times \text{collection time (h)}}$$

Water excretion fraction

$$= \text{urine vol. (ml/min)} \times \text{osmolar clearance}$$

Renal failure index

$$= \frac{\text{urine Na} \times \text{serum creatinine}}{\text{urine creatinine}}$$

Table 2.13 Renal function tests–differential diagnosis

	Pre-renal failure	Acute tubular necrosis
Urine specific gravity	> 1014	1005–1014
Urine osmolality	> 400	< 300
Urine Na	< 20	> 40
Urine urea	> 350 mmol/litre	< 175 mmol/litre
Urine/plasma creatinine	> 40	< 10
Urine/plasma urea	> 10	< 2
Urine/plasma osmolality	> 1.5	< 1.1
BUN/creatinine in serum	> 20	< 20
Sodium excretion fraction	< 1%	> 2%

Table 2.14 Types of casts

Cast	Condition
Hyaline	Pre-renal azotemia: obstructive uropathy
Red blood cells	Renal vascular diseases; glomerular disease
White blood cells	Interstitial nephritis
Pigmented cellular	Acute tubular necrosis

Table 2.15 Drugs excreted renally – dosage should be reviewed

Allopurinol	Carbenicillin	Flucytosine	Naproxen
Amikacin	Cefotaxime	Gentamicin	Netilmicin
Amoxycillin	Cefuroxime	Hydralazine	Phenobarbitone
Ampicillin	Cephalexin	Ibuprofen	Procainamide
Aspirin	Cimetidine	Kanamycin	Ranitidine
Atenolol	Diazoxide	Magnesium	Streptomycin
Azlocillin	Digoxin	Methicillin	Tetracylines
Captopril	Disopryamide	Metronidazole	Tobramycin
Carbamazepine	Ethacrinic acid	Mexiletine	Trimethoprim

Table 2.16 Drugs with little renal excretion – normal dosage may be safe in renal failure

Amphotericin	Erythromycin	Metoclopramide	Prednisolone
Chloramphenicol	Flucloxacillin	Metoprolol	Propranolol
Chlorpromazine	Flurazepam	Miconazole	Quinidine
Clindamycin	Heparin	Minoxidil	Rifampicin
Codeine	Hydrocortisone	Morphine	Salbutamol
Cortisone	Indomethacin	Nitroprusside	Theophylline
Dexamethasone	Labetalol	Pethidine	Tocainide
Diamorphine	Lignocaine	Phenytoin	Warfarin
Diazepam	Methylprednisolone	Prazosin	

Acid–base disturbances

Acidosis is the commonest such disturbance and, if metabolic, is the result of low cardiac output and lactic and pyruvic acid from the tissues. It worsens cardiac action further. Its treatment is the administration of sodium bicarbonate and sometimes tris-hydroxy-methyl-aminomethane (THAM) until the pH, bicarbonate and base excess are normal, plus the treatment of the predisposing circulatory insufficiency.

Formula for acidosis correction if pH < 7.2:

Required $NaHCO_3$:

$$(A) = \frac{BW \times base\ deficit}{5}$$

$$(B) = BW \times 0.4 \times (18 - real\ NaHCO_3)$$

Metabolic alkalosis occurs in about half of really ill postoperative patients at some stage, often associated with abnormally large potassium losses. The replacement of chloride to correct the acidosis and hypokalaemia is important. Nasogastric aspirations should be discontinued as soon as possible and hyperventilation avoided. Thiazide diuretics should be minimised and osmotic diuretics such as mannitol may be preferred if necessary in these cases. Potassium chloride to stop urinary hydrogen ion loss is the basis of treatment.

Nutritional aspects of cardiac surgery

Malnutrition (inadequate provision of substrates for growth, activity and tissue repair) causes loss of cellular mass (muscular and visceral), malfunction of vital organs, abnormal polymorphonuclear chemotaxis, dropping in the number of T cell rosettes, intracellular contraction, extracellular expansion and increased susceptibility to infection and delayed wound healing, as well as a higher incidence of respiratory failure secondary to muscular wasting.

The heart is, of course, affected by malnutrition, with deterioration of stroke volume, low cardiac output, ECG abnormalities, decreased oxygen consumption and myocardial atrophy. Chronic heart disease may itself lead to malnutrition from poor tissue perfusion, hypoxia and hypermetabolism, added to the lack of appetite caused by dyspnoea, hypomotility of the gastrointestinal tract, mental depression, distaste for food and lack of exercise.

The lung is also affected: atrophy of the respiratory muscles, deterioration in ventilatory mechanics, low vital capacity, depression of the hypoxic ventilatory response and respiratory failure.

Many patients with previous heart failure show cardiac cachexia, with no glycogen reserves in their tissues, especially the myocardium, the respiratory muscles and the liver. When they are subjected to cardiopulmonary bypass, they undergo massive metabolic changes: increased mobilisation of endogenous substrates and carbohydrate stores, hydrolysis of triglycerides, lysis of protein for gluconeogenesis and the effects of the hormones liberated during and after the operation.

Nutritional support may be offered by enteral and parenteral nutrition. The first is effective as long as the gastrointestinal tract is working normally. Unfortunately, in these patients with chronic malnutrition, there is atrophy of intestinal villi and poor absorption. Furthermore, the concentrations of some commercial compounds are high, the hyperosmolality causing diarrhoea. Parenteral nutrition, on the other hand, may overload the patient and is a possible source of infection from the catheter and the solutions.

Neurological problems

Coma is the unwelcome evidence of neurological damage of diffuse type resulting from cardiac surgery; its depth and associated neurological signs suggest the likely outcome. Meanwhile, treatment is directed at the prevention of adverse consequences. The airway should be secure, lack of respiratory drive and cough reflexes and power compensated for artificially in the routine way, and vasomotor instability watched for and treated according to the principles already mentioned, avoiding catecholamine-induced peripheral vasoconstriction and associated cerebral consequences.

Nutrition should be via a nasogastric tube as soon as possible, with high nutrition intravenous feeding until then. Care of pressure areas, catheterisation of the bladder, avoidance of corneal ulceration and suitable restraint to the restless patient are important.

Cultures should be taken regularly of sputum, urine and any areas of broken skin including the wound, and antibiotics immediately given as appropriate. Fits should be treated with phenytoin 200 mg stat and 50 mg 8-hourly intravenously with additional diazepam if necessary.

As soon as neurological damage is diagnosed, large doses of dexamethasone (10 mg i.v.) should be given, then 4 mg 6-hourly for three days to minimise the cerebral reaction. Oedema of the brain can also be reduced with diuretics – enough mildly to dehydrate the patient – and hyperosmolar colloidal infusions such as triple-strength plasma or human albumin. Mannitol, sucrose or hypertonic saline may pass into the brain and then worsen oedema after initially improving it, by taking water from the brain. Controlled hyperventilation and reduction of the body temperature in conjunction with a 'lytic cocktail' may improve the prospects for the brain cells.

Haematological problems

Postoperative bleeding is minimised by tidy surgery and ensuring a dry wound before closure, after as little bypass time as possible, in which as little transfused blood as possible has been used.

Patients with deficient clotting factors, especially with polycythaemia and those with a tendency to hypercoagulability and low cardiac output are more than normally prone to postoperative bleeding, while the likelihood of surgical bleeding is increased by connective tissue friability in such conditions as Marfan's syndrome.

Bleeding diseases like haemophilia, Christmas, abnormal platelets or abnormal capillaries should be diagnosed before surgery and treated. Operation should be delayed for two weeks after aspirin if possible.

Platelet defects, defibrination, fibrinolysis, persistence of heparin and shortness of factors V, VII, IX and X may develop during surgery. Full blood count, platelet count, prothrombin time (factors V, VII, X, II), kaolin–cephalin time (factors XII, XI, IX, VIII), bleeding time (platelets and capillary function), heparin–protamine titration (residual heparin), fibrinogen level and Fi test (fibrinolysis) help to identify causes of postoperative bleeding. While the tests are being done, replacement should be with fresh blood, which contains the factors V and VII absent from older blood, which can get very depleted when large transfusions are given. If the haemoglobin is normal, fresh frozen plasma is a good first line of plasma volume replacement for the same reason. If the tests show persistent heparin action, protamine should be given with further heparin titration control; intravascular coagulation producing defibrination is treated with heparin, and epsilon-aminocaproic acid (EACA) is the treatment of fibrinolysis, ensuring that heparin is given first, if fibrinolysis coexists with intravascular coagulation.

Low fibrinogen requires, of course, fibrinogen. Low prothrombin needs blood transfusion and vitamin K. Low platelets are supplemented with fresh blood platelet transfusion.

Massive transfusion should be of fresh blood, warm and compensated for with $CaCl_2$ (3.5 ml of 10% solution for every unit of blood), reopening when blood loss exceeds 300–400 ml per hour or when there is a suspicion of cardiac tamponade.

Pyrexia

Though early central pyrexia is usually the result of lowered cardiac output with peripheral vasospasm and failure to lose central heat to the periphery, late pyrexia is suggestive of infection (in the wound, urine, chest or, worst of all, the bloodstream from a prosthesis).

All should be sent for culture; infected wounds should be opened and drained. All intravenous cannulae should be checked for phlebitis (strict asepsis should always be observed in their management) and any evoking redness removed. The deep veins of the leg should be checked for tenderness. If all these investigations are negative, drugs should be discontinued one by one if possible and blood cultures can then be repeated in the absence of antibiotics, as well as blood count, film, Paul–Bunnell, cytomegalovirus, Australia antigen, antiheart antibodies, and other serology as indicated by local virology.

A diagnosis of 'post-cardiotomy syndrome' is one of exclusion of infection and, when arrived at, indicates aspirin therapy, or steroids if the first fails.

Liver failure

Peri-operative ischaemic hepatic damage is the likeliest cause of postoperative jaundice in those whose pre-operative hepatic function was normal, but other causes should be excluded.

Ischaemic damage of liver cells from low cardiac output produces a mixed obstructive and hepatocellular jaundice. There is also haemolysis of cells damaged by the heart–lung machine or the turbulence of paravalvular leaks, septal defects or malfunctioning prosthetic valves.

Jaundice is thus seen with multiorgan dysfunction: the sick-cell syndrome. The real culprit is the malfunctioning heart and its inadequate output.

There are some cases of fulminant liver failure in which encephalopathy is the most important manifestation. These cases can be classified into:

Grade I: Minor drowsiness; impaired concentration.
Grade II: Moderate drowsiness; confusion; disorientation.
Grade III: Severe drowsiness; stuporous; aggressive.
Grade IV: (a) Coma; response to pain.
              (b) Coma; no response to any stimuli.

In cardiac surgical patients this can present especially related to idiosyncratic drug reactions: allopurinol, monoamine oxidase inhibitors, sulphonamides, tetracycline, riboflavin, isoniazid, ketoconazole, phenytoin, and in paracetamol overdose.

Treatment in moderate cases is based on protein withdrawal, lactulose and neomycin. Also, to avoid gastrointestinal bleeding, H_2 antagonists are administered. Fluid balance must be checked even more carefully, avoiding saline solutions. Blood glucose is checked regularly.

When there is worsening of the clinical situation, each complication is treated on its merits. Thus cerebral oedema is managed with mannitol and ultrafiltration; renal failure with haemodialysis; hypoxia with physiotherapy and ventilation if required; haemorrhage with fresh frozen plasma, vitamin K and platelets; and so forth.

In summary, when the cardiac surgical patient has signs of hepatic dysfunction, the consequences must be treated. The liver needs adequate glucose and vitamins, and not too many fats, ethanol or hepatotoxic drugs or anaesthetic agents. Albumin may need to be supplemented intravenously, and coagulation must be checked, especially if the patient has to be on warfarin for a mechanical valve.

Neomycin may sterilise the gut and minimise portal venous bacteraemia, though the evidence for benefit was in dogs which normally have portal bacteraemia. Charcoal column haemo-dialysis or pig liver dialysis are desperate measures worthy of mention but probably not of action. Bowel washouts, oral protein restriction and neomycin may prevent the development of hepatic coma in toxic, pyrexial, profoundly generally ill patients. Hepatic transplantation is only worth considering for late, chronic hepatic failure.

If total parenteral nutrition is necessary in liver failure, solutions without aromatic aminoacids are mandatory, since aliphatic aminoacids can be metabolised peripherally.

Late postoperative management

After discharge from the intensive care ward, the return to twice daily check-overs by the house staff, twice weekly blood counts, electrolyte, prothrombin and enzyme assays, X-rays and electro-cardiogram, should be gradual, the frequency of testing reducing as the situation stabilises. Daily weighing should replace the scrupulous fluid balance charts of the ITU as a means of assessing fluid balance and the need for diuretics. A portable ECG eases the transition from ITU monitoring to 6-hourly TPR and BP charts.

All mechanical valve replacements should have anticoagulation. As soon as the drains are removed, therefore, the loading dose of warfarin is given. Evidence suggests the long-term coronary graft patency rate is favourably influenced by soluble aspirin 75 mg a day. An aspirin a day may help to prevent platelet thrombi forming on valves (which warfarin would not prevent), and aspirin/dipyridamole cover suffices for tissue valves.

Antibiotics are given prophylactically to open heart patients over surgery. When no prosthesis is implanted, these are only necessary over the three days or so when drips and drains are still installed, whereas they should be given for a fortnight with prostheses. Flucloxacillin provides cover against the commoner (oral) bacteria. The short-term, narrow spectrum policy minimises the risk of promoting multiresistant strains. Careful watch should be kept for fungal superinfection in sicker patients. Emphatic instruction should be given to all patients with prosthetic material implanted, to ensure that full antibiotic cover is given whenever any dental work is done or localised infections exist or urethral instrumentation performed.

Monitoring

The variety of type and complexity of equipment available for use in the Intensive Therapy Unit is wide and forever expanding, as is the growth in the electronics industry in general.

Although the equipment available would appear to be able to monitor, control and provide printed trend analysis for most physiological events, it is easy to forget that systems still depend on being set up correctly with proper application of electrodes, accurate calibrations of amplifiers and even secure connection of taps and tubing. Most problems encountered in the use of monitoring and assist equipment can be traced to simple errors in the initial setting-up period and it is always advisable at first to think of simple reasons why a machine may not be giving the expected results.

Electrocardiogram

The electrocardiogram is the basic signal displayed by a bedside monitor on an ITU to give warning of undesirable rhythms. The signal is easily obtained providing certain measures are carried out at the time of connecting patient to monitor, otherwise the information displayed may be misleading and prevent the correct use of alarm systems. In order that reliable heart rate alarms can be set or true arrhythmia analysis be performed, it is essential that the following points are observed.

Siting of electrodes

For correct processing of the ECG signal, a waveform must be presented to the monitor which shows an 'R wave' which is much larger than the 'T wave' in order that the monitor can distinguish the former for triggering the heart rate counter and provide an adequate synchronising signal for cardioversion or intra-aortic balloon pumping. It is also desirable that the displayed waveform clearly shows a 'P wave' for help in rhythm analysis. To obtain the above, preferred sites for attachment of electrodes are near the cardiac apex and at the upper sternum, although exact positioning will depend on the individual patient.

Application of electrodes

Pre-jelled adhesive electrodes are standard in most units and are simple and quick to apply, providing some skin preparation is used to reduce skin impedance for signal transmission and to provide a dry surface for good skin adhesion. Adequate preparation can usually be achieved by rubbing the skin with gauze or by use of the abrasive pad provided on most pre-jelled electrodes. Sometimes a spirit solution may be necessary, but if used this must be allowed to dry before the electrode is applied.

Monitoring problems

Heart rate alarms can often be falsely triggered by poor signal quality and this can be due to one of two causes. The first is an ECG signal containing excessive 'noise', which may be the result of poor electrode application, or of movement of the patient's cable with transmitted stress to the electrode connection. The latter is best minimised by taping the cable to the patient and it is good practice to do this routinely.

The second cause of monitoring problems is that of waveform shapes as indicated above. Low-amplitude QRS waveforms, broad RSR patterns of paced complexes may not present acceptable or consistent signals to the monitor and therefore time spent initially in obtaining optimal signals will prevent such confusion later.

Heart rate alarms which trigger repeatedly or rhythm analysers which give incorrect messages, all due to false information, are likely to be switched off permanently, with obvious hazardous implications.

Blood pressure

Arterial blood pressure can be monitored non-invasively but if continuous recordings of analysis of waveform shape is desired, together with left atrial, pulmonary arterial or central venous pressure display, then an invasive system is necessary.

Invasive pressure monitoring system

All necessary tubing for pressure monitoring is readily available in pre-packed sterile kits and even transducers can now be obtained as a disposable item, but understanding the basic principles of this technique is essential if meaningful results are to be obtained.

The standard transducer for invasive blood pressure monitoring is that of the strain-gauge type, whether it is disposable or re-usable. The operation of this device is based on the Wheatstone bridge principle, the circuitry being attached to a flexible diaphragm which separates the electronics from the fluid-filled tubing connected to the patient. Transmission of pressure waves along the tubing causes distortion of the diaphragm, which in turn varies the output from the bridge circuit in proportion to the applied pressure.

Transducer tubing criteria

To display and measure a waveform which contains minimal distortion, the transducer tubing system must follow certain criteria:

1. The transducer should have a low volume displacement and the tubing should be stiff-walled to prevent 'absorption' of the transmitted pressure wave; that is, the system should have a low compliance.
2. The tubing should be wide bore and as short as possible.
3. The system must be bubble-free and all connections tight. Plastic stopcocks readily 'hide' bubbles and must be carefully checked.

A bedside monitoring system capable of operating over a frequency range of 0–20 Hz (± 3 dB) will cause minimal distortion to the arterial waveform and will be satisfactory for routine requirements.

Setting-up system

Providing the correct tubing has been chosen and the system has been filled correctly, with the elimination of all bubbles, the monitor will require the zero and calibration points to be set.

With tap A closed to the patient and tap B open to atmosphere, the zero button on the monitor is pressed and the zero pressure allowed to register on the screen and meter display. Tap B is then closed to atmosphere and tap A opened to the monitoring line. This line can be used as a calibration line if it is held at a known height above the zero port (i.e. 68 cm = 50 mmHg) and is filled with fluid. The monitor calibration is adjusted if necessary.

The transducer is positioned with its zero port at the level of the patient's atria (4th intercostal space at the mid-axilla). If the position of the patient is changed after setting up, then the transducer level must be adjusted. The transducer position should be checked before pressure readings (particularly CVP and left atrial) are recorded on the patient's chart. If the transducer position is 10 cm below its recommended position, the displayed pressure reading will be 7.3 mmHg higher than its true value and conversely, if 10 cm above, will be 7.3 mmHg lower. If the venous pressure measurement line is used for drug infusion, then the infusion port must momentarily be closed to allow correct venous pressure to be recorded and its true waveform to be observed.

Measurement of pulmonary arterial and indirect left atrial pressure by Swan–Ganz technique

In cases where a direct left atrial line is not inserted during cardiac surgery, an alternative method for obtaining pulmonary arterial and left atrial pressure is that of using a balloon flotation (Swan–Ganz) catheter. This type of catheter is also obtainable with a distal thermistor for measuring cardiac output by the thermal dilution technique.

A size 7F thermal dilution catheter is introduced through an 8F sheath into a subclavian or jugular vein and advanced to the right atrium. If fluoroscopy is not available, the catheter tip position can be judged by reference to the markings on the catheter wall. The balloon is inflated with air to its recommended volume and the action of blood flow on the balloon, together with manipulation of the catheter, will direct the latter into the right ventricle and pulmonary artery. Monitoring of pressure waveforms via the distal lumen will indicate the chamber and vessel reached. Pulmonary arterial pressure will be observed as soon as the balloon passes the pulmonary valve and, as the catheter advancement is continued, a wedge position will be reached and the indirect left atrial waveform displayed on the monitor screen. The wedge pressure reading should be noted and the balloon deflated and the catheter secured proximally. Further inflation of the balloon to take recordings should be performed gradually to prevent damage to a small pulmonary artery branch, should the catheter tip have moved since its initial positioning. It may not be necessary fully to inflate the balloon to obtain an adequate wedge tracing. The catheter lumen is kept patent by use of a continuous flushing device.

To perform a thermal dilution measurement (Figure 2.2), a bolus (10 ml) of cold saline is injected rapidly through the proximal lumen of the catheter into the right atrium. The bolus will mix with and cool blood on its passage through the right heart and the resultant drop in temperature of the blood is measured by the distal thermistor in the pulmonary artery. The cardiac output can

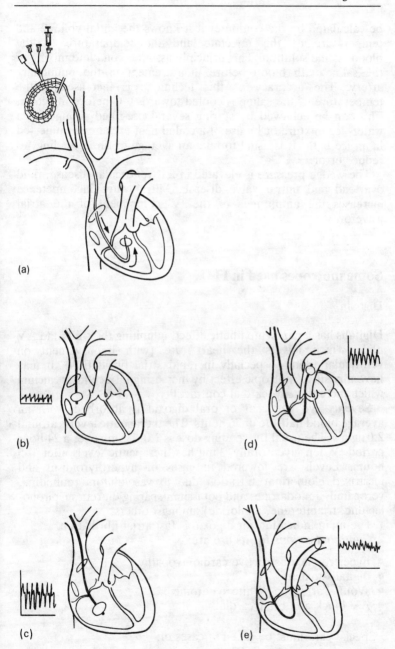

Figure 2.2 (*a*)–(*e*) Thermal dilution catheter for pressure and cardiac measurement

be calculated by the computer if it knows the initial volume and temperature of the injectate and the temperature of the blood–saline solution. This principle assumes complete mixing of the saline with blood before measurement in the pulmonary artery. The accuracy of this technique is increased if the temperature of the saline is cooled towards 0°C before injection. This can be achieved by storing several pre-filled syringes in a water–ice mixture or by use of a coiled heat exchanger immersed in an ice bath. It is usual to take an average of three readings to reduce error.

The wedge pressure is elevated in left ventricular disease, fluid overload and mitral valve disease. Mitral valve incompetence increases the amplitudes of the 'V' component of the atrial waveform.

Some inotropes used in ITU

Digoxin

Digitalis has a parasympathetic effect, inhibiting the sinus and AV node which lowers the heart rate (with improvement on ventricular filling, especially in rapid atrial fibrillation). It may have a positive inotropic effect by increasing intracellular calcium which increases myocardial contractility.

Seventy-five per cent of oral digoxin is absorbed, with an average blood half-life of 36 hours. The therapeutic level is around 2.0 ng/ml. The usual i.v. loading dose is 1.0–1.5 mg over a 24-hour period. When given orally, 1 mg has therapeutic levels after 1–5 hours. Levels are lowered in cases of hyperthyroidism and increased glomerular filtration due to vasodilators (quinidine, verapamil, amiodarone) and potassium-sparing diuretics (spirono-lactone, triamterene, amiloride) amongst others.

The main indication for digoxin is fast atrial fibrillation.
Contraindications for its use are:

• hypertrophic obstructive cardiomyopathy
• digitalis-toxicity
• Wolff–Parkinson–White syndrome
• AV block and bradycardia.

Special care must be taken in cases of:

• valvular stenosis

- hyperthyroidism
- acute myocardial infarction
- renal failure
- myocarditis
- precardioversion.

Digitalis toxicity usually presents in elderly patients with deteriorated renal function, chronic heart failure and pulmonary disease and is due to cellular overload with calcium, excessive vagal stimulation and depression of the conduction system. The factors which increase the risk of intoxication are divided into:

- pharmaceutical (excess dose)
- decreased volume of distribution (renal failure, hypo-thyroidism)
- decreased renal clearance (renal failure, quinidine, verapamil, amiodarone)
- decreased metabolic clearance (antibiotics, hepatic impair-ment).

Electrolyte changes can alter the effects of digoxin by sensitising to toxic ones (hypokalaemia, hypomagnesaemia), by increasing sensitivity to digitalis (hypercalcaemia) or by decreasing that sensitivity (hypocalcaemia). On the other hand, drugs that may alter the absorption of digoxin may decrease its levels (cholestyr-amine, kaolin, antacids, neomycin, rifampicin, cimetidine, hydra-lazine and sodium nitroprusside).

The main *symptoms* are:

- anorexia
- nausea
- vomiting
- diarrhoea
- fatigue
- confusion
- depression
- facial pain
- vertigo
- coloured vision
- palpitations
- arrhythmias
- syncope.

On examination the patient is usually bradycardic and sometime acutely ill, with signs of associated hypokalaemia. The direct cardiac effects may be classified into arrhythmias, heart block and worsening of heart failure. The ECG may show:

- heart block
- bigeminy
- atrial tachycardia
- AV junctional escape beats
- ventricular tachycardia (sometimes).

Treatment includes withdrawing digitalis and giving potassium (intravenous in severe cases: 0.5 mEq/min, checking the potassium at least half-hourly; orally in stable patients: 50–80 mEq in divided doses). Drugs that may elevate digoxin levels are also withdrawn (verapamil, quinidine). In multiple ventricular ectopics, lignocaine is given at usual doses. Also, phenytoin may reverse the heart block. In cases of severe heart block a pacemaker is indicated.

Dopamine

This catecholamine-like agent is a noradrenaline precursor and it also releases noradrenaline from stores in the nerve endings of the heart, activating beta-1 receptors which cause inotropic and chronotropic effects of the heart, as well as coronary vasodilatation. Also, by its action on beta-2 receptors in other tissues, it causes peripheral vasodilatation. The direct action over DA_1 receptors leads to renal vasodilatation and diuresis. The action on DA_2 receptors inhibits noradrenaline release, leading to further peripheral vasodilatation. At high doses, the action of alpha receptors leads to general vasoconstriction.

Dopamine is indicated in cardiogenic shock, refractory heart failure, low cardiac output after open cardiothoracic surgery, septic shock and in early states of renal failure. It is contraindicated in ventricular arrhythmias.

The usual dose is 2–10 µg/kg/min (see p. 63).

Dobutamine

Acts more specifically over beta-1 adrenergic receptors, causing inotropic and chronotropic effects. It does not affect dopamine receptors. The effects on beta-1 and alpha receptors are weak. It is used in low cardiac output following myocardial infarction and cardiac surgery.

The usual dose is 2–10 µg/kg/min (see p. 63).

Adrenaline

Its beta stimulation cardiac effects are positively inotropic and chronotropic, as well as causing peripheral and coronary vasodilatation. The alpha effects cause vasoconstriction. It is used particularly in emergency situations, or when other inotropes have failed in cases of severe low cardiac output syndrome.

The dose is 0.02–0.2 µg/kg/min.

Noradrenaline

By stimulating beta-1 receptors on the heart, it increases the heart rate, AV conduction and enhances myocardial contractility.

Alpha stimulation causes peripheral vasoconstriction and raises the blood pressure. The action over beta-2 receptors causes peripheral vasodilatation and bronchodilatation. Nevertheless, these beneficial effects on the failing heart are vitiated by its arrhythmogenic effects, as well as by the increasing myocardial oxygen demand.

Isoprenaline

This synthetic sympathometic amine has nearly pure beta-adrenergic activity, increasing the cardiac rate and contractility, and reducing the afterload by peripheral vasodilatation.

The usual dose is 0.02–02 µg/kg/min.

Ventricular support (mechanical)

Balloon counter-pulsation

This is a technique of providing temporary mechanical assistance to the distressed heart, first proposed by Moulopoulos in 1962 and further developed by Kantrowitz in 1967.

Objectives

1. To reduce myocardial oxygen demand by reducing the work required of the left ventricle to eject blood into the aorta.
2. To increase coronary arterial blood flow during diastole (80% of coronary flow occurs during this part of the cardiac cycle).

Indications

1. *Cardiogenic shock:* pump failure – insufficient cardiac output despite adequate venous return, ventilation, fluids, acid–base balance and cardiotonics. Such a patient would exhibit an increased cardiac rate (110–140 b.p.m.), a systolic blood pressure < 80 mmHg, urine output < 20 ml per hour, and may be confused and disorientated.
2. *Unstable angina:* patients with precordial pain at rest due to poor myocardial blood flow may be stabilised by the IABP technique, thus preventing myocardial infarction.
3. *Post-infarction ventricular septal defect:* results in the shunting of blood from the left to the right heart. This effect can be reduced by reducing left ventricular afterload.
4. *Post-cardiopulmonary bypass:* following cardiac surgery, the heart may sometimes require assistance by the intra-aortic balloon pump in order to wean the patient from the cardiopulmonary bypass apparatus.

Method

A plastic catheter, of 3–4 mm diameter, is introduced into the femoral artery and advanced through the abdominal and the thoracic aorta until its distal tip is just below the level of the left subclavian artery. Moulded around the distal end of the catheter is a 40 ml (typical adult size) balloon which is 28 cm in length and 1.5 cm in diameter. Positioning of the balloon is determined by measurement of the catheter externally against the patient's body prior to insertion, or by means of radiographic screening if available.

Insertion of catheter

1. *Surgical (a).* The common femoral artery is exposed and two purse-string snares are placed on its front. The catheter is measured externally against the patient's body and a marker noted on the catheter at a point level with the proposed entry to the artery. The balloon is collapsed by the creation of a vacuum within it and the catheter is introduced into the artery while this is controlled. The upper control is released while the balloon is passed gently upwards until the distal tip is positioned below the left subclavian artery. The purse-string sutures are tied and the wound closed around the catheter after use of an antibiotic spray. A formal closure of the artery is required when the catheter is removed, accompanied by pro- and retrograde embolectomy catheterisation.

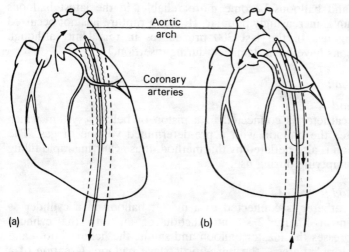

Figure 2.3 Balloon operation: (*a*) deflation – systole; (*b*) inflation – diastole

2. *Surgical (b)*. The catheter may be introduced via a synthetic graft sewn to the artery wall.
3. *Surgical (c)*. Should the common iliac or aorta be too atheromatous to allow free passage of the balloon, it is possible to introduce the catheter through the anterior aortic arch. The balloon is then advanced pro-gradely down the descending aorta and positioned in the thoracic aorta as for the retrograde route, the proximal end of the catheter this time being brought out through the chest wall.
4. *Percutaneous*. Entry may be made into the femoral artery by the Seldinger technique. This method is more often used with a double lumen catheter and the aid of a guide-wire through the central monitoring lumen, but can be used with single lumen catheters through the introducer sheath provided with balloon kits. On removal of a percutaneous system, the balloon is deflated and the sheath and catheter are withdrawn together; pressure is applied until the site is dry.

Priming of the catheter

The catheter, balloon and any extension tubing are primed with helium, whose virtue is its low density and hence viscosity, or carbon dioxide, whose virtue is its ability to dissolve in blood should the balloon rupture during use. As the catheter lumen is less and balloons become more reliable, in the latest balloons helium is increasingly popular. (Balloon rupture has not occurred during use in the last 300 procedures in this Unit, although balloons have been damaged during insertion.)

Inflation

Method A

The catheter is connected to a piston or bellows system which inflates the balloon with a pre-determined volume of gas. The balloon is also deflated by this method, thus achieving rapid filling and emptying during use.

Method B

The catheter is connected to a master balloon in a cylinder as shown in Figure 2.3. Introduction of air into the cylinder compresses the master balloon and shunts the helium into – and therefore inflates – the intra-aortic slave balloon. Creation of a vacuum in the cylinder expands the master balloon and thus deflates the slave balloon.

Control

Electrocardiogram

The 'R wave' of the signal is used as a trigger for deflation of the balloon to correspond with the instant of ventricular rapid contraction, and the reflation is set manually for the optimal subsequent time, ideally as the aortic valve closes after systole.

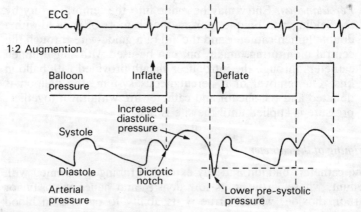

Figure 2.4 Optimal balloon timing

Arterial pressure
The upstroke of the arterial pressure waveform can be used as a trigger source and may be useful where the ECG signal is of poor quality or irregular in shape.

Problems

1. Loss of trigger signal because:
   (a) ECG is too small;
   (b) ECG shape is 'abnormal'.

   To rectify:
   (a) increase ECG size with gain control;
   (b) change polarity of sensing;
   (c) change position of electrodes;
   (d) use pressure trigger.

2. Irregular trigger due to:
   (a) as above;
   (b) ectopic beats or arrhythmias;
   (c) demand-pacing.

   To rectify:
   (a) increase pacing rate or try pressure trigger or use pacer reject trigger if available.

3. Poor augmentation due to:
   (a) incorrect timing settings (Figure 2.5);
   (b) incorrect balloon volume setting;
   (c) poorly positioned balloon;
   (d) kinked catheter, tight fixing suture;
   (e) sheath obstructing balloon-inflation.

   To rectify:
   (a) adjust;
   (b) adjust;
   (c) adjust if possible;
   (d) straighten catheter, release suture;
   (e) withdraw sheath.

4. Ischaemic leg – to rectify:
   Remove catheter as soon as possible or introduce new one in other leg if patient still dependent; scrupulous Fogarty catheterisation of the femoral vessels is even more important than usual.

ECG Trigger

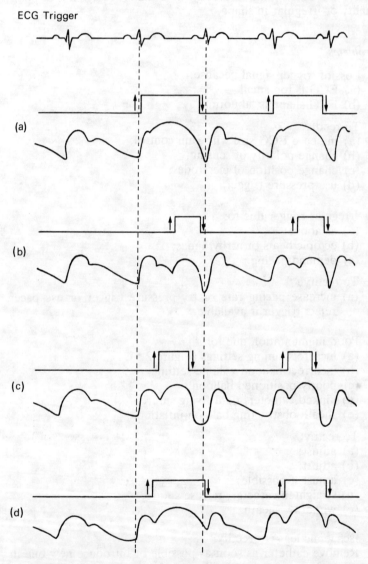

Figure 2.5 Incorrect timing setting: (*a*) inflation too early – impedes ejection; (*b*) inflation too late – loss of augmentation; (*c*) deflation too early – loss of augmentation; (*d*) deflation too late – impedes ejection

Left ventricular assist devices

When even balloon counterpulsation fails to provide an adequate cardiac output, the whole action of the left ventricle can be substituted by a pump. This should only be done if either the ventricle promises to recover its contractility or if cardiac transplantation is a valid proposition.

Either with the patient heparinised, or using a heparin-bonded circuit, a cannula is introduced into the left atrium at thoracotomy and blood pumped by a centrifugal pump into an artery, usually the femoral.

An alternative, new device is a transfemoral catheter containing a small propeller, which is passed through the aortic valve and pumps blood from the left ventricle into the aorta beyond the aortic valve, which closes round the conducting pathway from the propeller.

Surgery in ischaemic heart disease

The results of surgery for ischaemic heart disease have largely standardised to an operative mortality of less than 2%; a peri-operative myocardial infarction rate of less than 5%; a graft patency of more than 90% in the first years, and similar survival rates in that period.

The main *indications* for surgery in coronary artery disease are:

1. Severe obstructive disease with incapacitating symptoms and poor response to medical treatment.
2. Severe left main stem obstruction.
3. Coronary disease and ventricular arrhythmias.
4. Coronary obstruction with associated surgical heart disease.
5. Post-infarction complications (ventricular septal rupture, papillary muscle dysfunction or rupture, ventricular aneurysm) and active residual coronary disease.
6. Unstable angina.
7. Evolving myocardial infarction treated by thrombolysis but relapsing.
8. Post-infarction angina.

The main *risk factors* are:

- age
- sex (female)
- left main stem obstruction
- poor ventricular function

- severe pulmonary disease
- associated fatal disease (cancer).

Contraindications to surgery may be summarised as:

- advanced heart failure with pulmonary hypertension and poor ejection fraction
- advanced pulmonary disease
- poor run-off in distal coronary vessels.

Complications of coronary artery disease are also amenable to surgical treatment. These include:

1. *Ventricular septal rupture.* The prognosis of early operation is still very poor and if the patient can be supported medically (including intra-aortic balloon) for two weeks, the survival rate improves substantially. This 'improvement' may be spurious, and the result of self-selection of better-risk cases.
2. *Mitral valve insufficiency.* The same applies regarding timing for surgery. Nevertheless, in both situations the only definitive treatment is surgical.
3. *Ventricular aneurysm.* Operation is indicated if the aneurysm is causing heart failure, angina, ventricular arrhythmias and systemic emboli.

When intracoronary thrombolysis has been attempted unsuccessfully or if intraluminal balloon coronary dilatation is complicated by acute coronary obstruction during the procedure, coronary bypass grafting is performed urgently.

Complications after coronary arterial surgery

The most important complication after bypass surgery is peri-operative myocardial infarction, which may be pre-, intra- or postoperative.

Pre-operative infarction may be caused by sudden cessation of medical treatment or by hypoxia, particularly in the anaesthetic room.

Intra-operative infarction is generally due to poor myocardial protection and to failures in surgical technique.

Postoperative infarction is usually due to occlusion of a graft or inadequate revascularisation.

If a correctable cause is detected, the treatment must be carried out promptly, especially if acute ischaemia is proved immediately after surgery. Otherwise, medical treatment for ischaemia is restarted.

Other complications include low cardiac output, cardiac tamponade and bleeding (see p. 58 et seq.).

Valve surgery

Varieties of prosthetic valves

Mechanical

- Starr Edwards (SE)
- Bjork Shiley (BSM)
- Lillehei Kaster (LLK)
- Omniscience (OMI)
- Medtronics (MED)
- St Jude Medical (SJM)
- Duromedics (DM)
- Carbomedics (CM)

Silastic-balled valve
The original design – mainly Starr Edwards which still is the basic standard. Better 'curing' of the silastic has prevented its deterioration.

Disc valve
The discs are now made of pyrolite, which is almost diamond-hard carbon and has a negative surface charge. The differences are in the mode of retention of the disc, which can rotate and thus wears evenly. The different mounts permit various degrees of opening. Ninety degrees would be the ideal as then a well-streamlined disc would be sideways on to the bloodstream and would provoke the least turbulence. Closure from this angle is unfortunately too slow and associated with an undue amount of regurgitation.

While silastic balls shed any clot that forms on them, disc valves would more likely accumulate the clot as a pannus which eventually traps the disc, so these valves are less obstructive to flow than ball valves, less likely to produce emboli but more likely to become 'frozen' by pannus. They include the Bjork Shiley, Lillehei Kaster, Narco, and Hall Medtronics.

Double hemidisc valves
These have the advantages of more laminar flow as the centrally hinged discs open fully and are side-on to the fastest part of the stream. They are all-pyrolite (including the annulus) so are even

less thrombogenic than pyrolite-disc-only valves. They have not been available as long as the other varieties so their long-term performance is not yet perfectly known. They are, however, the most promising hardware option. Examples: St Jude, Carbomedics.

The most important disadvantage of mechanical valves is the need for anticoagulation for their thrombogenicity. Also, their audibility might make them poorly tolerated by the patient.

Biological

- Homograft
- Carpentier Edwards Porcine (CE)
- Carpentier Edwards Pericardial (CEP)
- Carpentier Edwards Supra-annular (CES)
- Ionescu Shiley (IS)
- Mitral Medical Pericardial (MMP)
- Wessex Porcine (WP)
- Liotta (LI)
- Hancock (HA)
- Killingbeck (KLK)
- Tascon (TAC)

Human valves
The original replacement for the aortic valve was human aortic valve. Nowadays, inserted after less than three weeks and kept in antibiotic medium, their performance is good, but skill and experience are necessary for insertion, which makes their use confined to centres where the necessary enthusiasm exists.

Porcine valves
These are commercially available sewn to manufactured mounting rings which make them affixable by the same techniques as all manufactured valves. They include Hancock, Liotta, Carpentier Edwards and Wessex. The variations are those of fixation and mount shape. All are fixed at low tension which keeps the collagen more 'crinkly' and flexible.

Pericardial valves
This pattern is biological in that it is glutaraldehyde-fixed pericardium but handcrafted into cusp form with some resultant benefit to haemodynamic performance. The Ionescu Shiley, Mitral Medical Pericardial and Carpentier Pericardial are the main brands of this type.

All these biological valves are minimally thrombogenic and can thus be used without anticoagulants in those patients wishing to have pregnancies or to boldly go where no anticoagulant supervision is available. Their durability is the unknown fact – so far it appears that they will last between 5 and 10 years.

Mitral stenosis

This is always acquired from rheumatic disease and presents with dyspnoea, pulmonary oedema, arrhythmias or embolism.

Medical treatment is based on diuretics, sodium restriction, digoxin, beta blockers and treatment of complications (arrhythmias, peripheral embolism, haemoptysis, infection).

Surgery is indicated if the stenosis is severe, in the presence of pulmonary hypertension (critical diameter less than $1.5\,cm^2$) or if there is heavy calcification or symptoms of IIb or greater limitation. Commissurotomy is indicated in non-calcified pure mitral stenosis. Otherwise mitral valve replacement is performed, with a mechanical valve unless the patient is old, if pregnancy is expected or if anticoagulation is contraindicated, when a bioprosthetic valve is inserted.

Mitral incompetence

This is the most common valve lesion and may be primary (rheumatic fever, bacterial endocarditis, chordal or papillary muscle damage or flailing of cusp) or functional, secondary to aortic valve disease or cardiomyopathy.

Once the cause has been controlled, treatment with vasodilators (hydralazine, captopril, prazosin) in order to reduce the afterload, as well as diuretics, digoxin and inotropics if the patient is in heart failure, may suffice. Prophylaxis for infective endocarditis is important, particularly when dental procedures or surgery are anticipated, or active infections occur.

Operation is indicated in refractory heart failure and when other surgical heart diseases are present (coronary artery disease).

Aortic stenosis

Aortic stenosis may be congenital, degenerative or inflammatory. Its symptoms may start late in the course of the disease, but after the first episode of angina, syncope, dyspnoea or heart failure, death will come in 50% within 2 years.

The treatment is mechanical correction. It is conservative (surgical or percutaneous valvuloplasty) in congenital aortic stenosis or in non-calcified disease. Otherwise aortic valve replacement is mandatory. A gradient greater than 30 mmHg and a valve orifice smaller than 1 cm^2 indicates significant stenosis.

Almost any substitute valve performs well in the aortic position but if the annulus is small a double hemi-disc valve will perhaps give a small gradient. If anticoagulation is contraindicated a bioprosthetic valve is used.

Aortic incompetence

The main problem here is left ventricular volume overload with congestive heart failure.

Medical treatment should suffice provided there is not progressively increasing heart size or ST/T wave changes suggesting 'strain'.

Emergency surgery is indicated in acute incompetence due to infective endocarditis, particularly if vegetations or aortic root abscesses are present; also, if pulmonary oedema, septal involvement by the infection (heart block), renal failure or fungal endocarditis are diagnosed.

Tricuspid valve disease

This is generally secondary to mitral or aortic valve disease. Nevertheless, it can be affected by intravenously introduced endocarditis, rheumatic fever and carcinoid syndrome. When advanced or organic, severe right heart failure is present.

It is best assessed during operation as it is very rare for the tricuspid valve to fail primarily. A surgical 'rule-of-finger' is that, if the cusps are palpable with the exploring finger prior to cannulation for cardiopulmonary bypass, then the tricuspid will not regain competence with the correction of the primary left heart haemodynamic problem. Annuloplasty or replacement will thus be required.

Problems associated with valve surgery

In *closed mitral valvotomy* the main problem is thromboembolism. If the valve is calcified or a clot is found in the atrium, the procedure should be abandoned for an open valvotomy. Other possible problems are:

- bleeding from ventricular or atrial incisions
- severe regurgitation from excessive tension and cusps tearing
- incomplete valvotomy (suggested by low cardiac output and pulmonary oedema in the postoperative period).

Open mitral valve repair could be complicated by:

- valve damage (dilated ring, cusp damage or ruptured chordae)
- air embolism
- thromboembolism.

Mitral valve replacement can cause severe problems when the prosthesis is attached to an incompletely prepared valve ring or one too attenuated by excessive calcium removal. Other possible problems include:

- imperfect resection of the sub-valvular apparatus (too little: valvular jam; too much: ventricular perforation)
- paravalvular leak
- disruption of the atrioventricular junction (generally lethal and resulting from over-excision of the mitral valve ring, deep sutures, too large prosthesis or excessive surgical lifting)
- damage to the aortic valve
- heart block
- damage to the circumflex coronary artery by over-deep sutures.

Aortic valve replacement may cause:

- calcium embolism
- paravalvular leak
- bleeding from the aorta
- heart failure due to intraoperative ischaemic cardiac damage
- valve malfunction
- heart block.

Tricuspid valve replacement may be complicated by heart block due to the proximity of its septal leaflet to the bundle of His; also, thrombosis and refractory right heart failure.

Some *complications* related to valve surgery are:

1. Post-perfusion syndrome (2–8 weeks after surgery, presenting with fever, splenomegaly, lymphocytosis and neutropenia).
2. Post-pericardiotomy syndrome (polyserositis 4 weeks after the operation, presenting with temperature, pleuritis, myalgias, leukocytosis and pericarditis).
3. Blood trauma (mainly by mechanical valves in the aortic position) with haemolysis and anaemia.

4. Thrombosis, mostly associated with mechanical valves, may cause severe valve malfunction and systemic or pulmonary embolism.
5. Prosthetic endocarditis presents as sepsis, embolism and heart failure.
6. Valve dysfunction or perivalvular or valvular leak may lead to cardiac failure.

   Later complications are:

- calcification
- degeneration
- tearing of cusps in tissue valves
- adverse effects of anticoagulants and antiplatelet therapy
- late thrombosis or embolism in mechanical valves.

Cardiac transplantation

The main indication for cardiac transplantation is advanced terminal cardiac disease classified as NYHA 4, without the alternative of conventional medical or surgical treatment, and with a mortality higher than 90% per year if transplantation is not carried out. Any cardiac condition might cause this advanced state, amongst others:

- cardiomyopathies
- ischaemic disease
- valvular disease
- myocarditis
- non-malignant cardiac tumours
- some congenital heart diseases
- coronary embolism
- cardiac trauma.

   Contraindicatons to the procedure are:

- intractable high pulmonary vascular resistance (more than 6 units Wood or 600 dyn s cm^{-5})
- malignant disease
- active infection
- insulin-dependent diabetes mellitus
- severe hepatic dysfunction
- advanced renal failure
- recent pulmonary embolism
- collagen diseases

- severe peripheral vascular disease
- cardiac cachexia
- age more than 55 years
- social or family instability
- severe psychiatric problems.

In general, any disease or situation that may risk the procedure should be ruled out. Concurrent pulmonary, renal or hepatic transplantation may now permit the reduction of some contraindications.

The *donor* is selected taking into account:

- proved brain-death
- age less than 40 years
- absence of previous heart disease, or:
- hypertension, or:
- cardiac trauma, or:
- prolonged hypotension or long periods of cardiac massage
- normal electrocardiogram
- good cardiac output and low doses of inotrope to maintain haemodynamic stability.

Also, the donor should be within 20% of the recipient's body weight. The ischaemic time from the aortic cross-clamping must not exceed 4 hours.

Pre-operative laboratory studies (obviously after a complete clinical examination) are:

- full blood count
- coagulation screen
- blood group
- antibody screen
- urea
- electrolytes
- creatinine
- liver function tests
- Australia antigen
- serum uric acid
- autoantibodies (antinuclear, DNA antibodies, rheumatoid factor and others)
- immunoglobulin levels
- viral screen
- fasting blood glucose
- fasting lipids
- cholesterol
- cardiac enzymes

- urinalysis
- chest X-ray
- ECG
- echocardiogram
- tissue typing (lymphocyte cross-match, lymphocytotoxic antibodies).

Four hours before the operation the first dose of oral cyclosporine (4–8 mg/kg according to creatinine clearance) is given.

Intravenous flucloxacillin (2 g) is injected in the anaesthetic room, before inserting the lines. Also, if antithymocytic globulin is indicated, this is started at 30 ml/h (10 mg/kg diluted in 125 ml normal saline). Every blood product must be previously tested for CMV.

On bypass, the flow is kept low until rewarming, when it comes to 3.0–3.5 litres/min and a mean arterial pressure of 60 mmHg. Fifteen minutes prior to aortic cross-clamp removal, isoprenaline is started at 3 µg/kg/min, dopamine at 3 µg/kg/min, sodium nitroprusside at 10 µg/kg/min and adrenaline if the case requires it.

Once off bypass, methylprednisolone (500 mg i.v.), frusemide (20 mg i.v.), flucloxacillin (1 g), calcium chloride (10 mmol) and mannitol (25 ml mannitol 25% over 25 min) are administered.

Postoperatively a strict protocol is followed:

- Reverse barrier nursing, early extubation, early removal of central catheters and early mobilisation.
- Cyclosporin: 4–8 mg/kg/day, according to serum levels, in order to keep them around 350–450 ng/ml for the first 6 weeks and between 150–250 ng/ml afterwards. The doses are divided in two.
- Azathioprine (Imuran): 4 mg/kg starting dose, and 1–3 mg/kg/day afterwards, to keep the white blood count between 5000 and 8000/mm^3.
- Methylprednisolone: 500 mg i.v. once the patient is off bypass and then 125 mg i.v. 8-hourly for 36 hours.
- Prednisolone: is started 48 hours after the transplant, at 0.5 mg/kg/day the first day, reducing by 0.2 mg daily to reach a final dose of 0.2 mg/kg/day.

Rejection is detected by endomyocardial biopsy, which is done weekly for the first 6 weeks, fortnightly for the next 6 weeks, monthly for the next 3 months and every 3 months afterwards. If rejection is detected, this is treated on its merits by increasing cyclosporin or Imuran; if severe, with methylprednisolone pulse therapy (1 g daily for 3 days); if the results are not satisfactory or if rejection is severe, antithymocytic globulin at 7 mg/kg i.v. infusion over 6 hours, twice a day for 14 days. If rejection occurs later, the doses of prednisolone are increased accordingly.

Infection must be treated aggressively, studying the offending microorganism and with specific antibiotics for it.

Aortic aneurysms, dissection and peripheral vascular matters

Aneurysms of the thoracic aorta

Aneurysmal dilatation of the aorta is nowadays most commonly due to atherosclerosis (descending thoracic aorta) or cystic medial necrosis, with or without stigmata of Marfan's syndrome (ascending aorta). Syphilitic aneurysms, however, are still encountered and false aneurysms after non-penetrating chest trauma may present some time after the event. Dissecting aneurysms and traumatic aneurysms are discussed elsewhere.

Clinical features

The diagnosis of aortic aneurysm is usually suspected from the radiological findings on a chest radiograph, performed for one of the following reasons:

1. *Pressure on adjacent structures.* Such symptoms are legion and include dysphagia, SVC obstruction, stridor, Horner's syndrome and phrenic or recurrent laryngeal nerve palsy.
2. *Cardiac failure.* Dilatation of the ascending aorta can cause aortic valve dysfunction with aortic regurgitation.
3. *Pain,* particularly in the back, can be a feature, predominantly of descending thoracic aneurysms. Erosion of vertebral bodies may be evident on a lateral chest radiograph.
4. *Rupture.* By the time a thoracic aneurysm has ruptured it is usually fatal. Clinical features depend on the structure involved and include massive haematemesis (oesophagus), cardiac tamponade (pericardial activity), haemothorax (pleural cavity) and very rarely externally via an aortocutaneous fistula.
5. *Symptomless abnormality* found on incidental chest X-ray.

Investigation

The diagnosis is usually suspected on the basis of a chest radiograph performed in the course of investigation of one of the above clinical situations. Further evaluation is by one or more of the following definitive investigations.

Ultrasonography. Two-dimensional echocardiography can be useful in the diagnosis and assessment of ascending aortic aneurysms but is less useful in the regions of the arch and aortic isthmus. Full assessment of the thoracic aorta is therefore limited.

CT scanning, particularly in conjunction with intravenous contrast, is of great benefit both in establishing the diagnosis and in assessing the extent of aortic involvement. It has the benefit of being non-invasive and is therefore of particular value in repeated serial examinations.

Aortography is well established and is the 'gold standard'. Digital subtraction techniques are being used with increasing frequency and satisfactory aortic imaging can be achieved with central venous injection rather than by direct arterial injection. At present however, intra-arterial cannulation remains the norm. The invasive nature of aortography with the attendant risks limits its usefulness in serial investigation.

Indications for surgery

Operative management is generally indicated where the aneurysm is symptomatic (see above). In cases of rupture, if the patient is *in extremis,* it may be decided that surgery is not the most appropriate course.

Where the aneurysm is discovered on an incidental chest X-ray, the decision to operate is most difficult. In general terms, aneurysms of greater than 6 cm diameter are best managed surgically. Asymptomatic aneurysms less than 6 cm are probably best managed by repeat imaging, CT scanning being the investigation of choice. Enlargement of the aneurysm on serial investigation should be considered an indication for operation. This may be prevented by strict reduction of the systolic blood pressure, and especially the rate of rise of pressure, with beta-blocking drugs.

Operative management

This is best discussed with reference to the different regions of aorta involved – ascending aorta, descending aorta and aortic arch. Replacement of more than one of these segments is rarely necessary. Surgery on the arch is associated with a higher mortality and morbidity and should not be undertaken unless absolutely necessary. Aneurysmal dilatation of the arch is not uncommon, particularly in atheromatous disease, but surgery on the most dilated segment of aorta, ascending or descending, usually suffices.

Ascending aortic aneurysms

These are approached by median sternotomy using cardiopulmonary bypass. It is usually possible to site the aortic cannula distal to the aneurysm but where this is not possible, arterial return is achieved via femoral arterial cannulation. The aorta is clamped distal to the aneurysm and the heart arrested with a cardioplegic solution. Some, however, favour the use of continuous coronary perfusion. Where the aortic valve is normal a tube graft of Dacron is inserted. In the presence of aortic regurgitation, the valve is replaced (or less commonly repaired). Then the aneurysm is dealt with by a supracoronary tube graft. Alternatively, it may be necessary to replace the valve and ascending aorta with a valved conduit, with reimplantation of the coronary arteries.

Descending aortic aneurysms

As in dissecting aneurysms, a tube graft of 'Dacron' is inserted via a posterolateral thoracotomy. Rarely the graft may be required to be anastomosed in the abdomen across the diaphragm, perhaps in conjunction with more distal extension to the iliofemoral segment. There are several methods of achieving distal perfusion, the main concern being spinal cord ischaemia.

1. *Cross clamping of the aorta.* Many surgeons advocate the use of a 'simple' aortic clamping to accomplish the insertion of a tube graft and maintain this technique is safe with cross-clamp times of up to 30 minutes. This obviously involves a degree of speed. One possible adjunct is to monitor aortic pressure distal to the clamp.
2. *Heparin-bonded shunts* can be inserted into the distal aorta from either the apex of the LV, LA appendage or aorta proximal to the aneurysm. It gives the advantage of distal aortic perfusion without the need for full systemic heparinisation.
3. *Partial cardiopulmonary bypass,* either femorofemoral with oxygenator or LA–femoral vein with pump can be used. Although allowing distal perfusion, this carries the risks of both systemic heparinisation and bypass.

All descending thoracic repairs result in upper body hypertension and require expert anaesthesia to control this.

Arch aneurysms

These are approached by median sternotomy with femoral arterial return. Deep hypothermia with low flow and low pressure perfusion is used. Once the transverse arch is opened, a tube graft is inserted from within the lumen; openings are then made to accommodate the origins of the head and neck vessels. Very rarely one or more head and neck vessels may require replacement using a composite tube graft.

Complications

1. Mortality: isolated replacement of ascending or descending aorta carries a mortality risk of up to 10%. Involvement of the arch increases this to the order of 20%.
2. Paraplegia.
3. Stroke.

Summary

The main points of contention are:

1. Management of the asymptomatic aneurysm.
2. Protection of the spinal cord during descending aortic replacement. Each method of dealing with the distal aortic perfusion has its adherents. No consistently reliable method has been demonstrated however. In general terms, those units managing a small number of cases should probably employ one of the shunt or bypass methods.

Acute dissection of the aorta

Early diagnosis of this condition is essential and dependent on maintaining a high index of clinical suspicion in every case of chest pain and undiagnosed shock.

The main differential diagnosis is myocardial infarction. The pain of aortic dissection is classically described as 'tearing' in nature. It is often posterior. Many patients have a history of previous hypertension and may be hypertensive on admission, although clammy and peripherally vasoconstricted. Clinical signs include diminished or absent limb-pulses, stroke and paraplegia. When the ascending aorta is involved and the aortic valve or annulus affected, auscultatory signs of aortic regurgitation may be present.

Chest X-rays show widening of the mediastinum and perhaps left pleural effusion. ECG findings are not specific. Acute changes of myocardial infarction should be sought in order to exclude this as a diagnosis. However, when the coronary ostia are involved in the dissection (usually the right), the two conditions may become very difficult to differentiate. The definitive investigation is aortography, with or without digital substraction. It demonstrates the extent of the dissection and the site of intimal tearing. Ultrasonography and CT scanning can be useful in expert hands.

There are several recognised classifications of aortic dissection. One of them comes from Stanford and is based on the extent of aortic involvement rather than the anatomical site of the tear, which has important surgical implications.

- *Type A* refers to dissections where the ascending aorta is involved, regardless of the site of the intimal tear.
- *Type B* involves only the descending aorta.

Management

At present acute dissections are best managed by surgery once the diagnosis has been established.

Pre-operative management includes:

- adequate venous access with central venous cannulation if possible
- adequate pain relief
- oxygen therapy and maintenance of airway
- cross matching of at least 6 units of blood
- arterial line for blood pressure monitoring
- insertion of urinary catheter
- control of blood pressure. The systolic BP is best kept around 100 mmHg to minimise the risk of further dissection. Although there are advantages to beta blockade, as reduction of the rate of rise of pressure and the peak systolic pressure provides optimal protection from further dissection, in practice controlled hypotension is often achieved by nitroprusside infusion.

Type A dissections are approached via median sternotomy. Cardiopulmonary bypass is used. If no healthy ascending aorta is available for cannulation, arterial return is via a femoral arterial cannula. Once on bypass with systemic hypothermia, the aorta is clamped and the heart arrested with intracoronary cardioplegia and topical cooling. The aorta is opened and the site of intimal tear identified.

The aim of surgery is to resect the portion of aorta containing the tear, ensuring this resected area is as short as possible. End-to-end anastomosis is rarely possible and the interposition of a Dacron tube graft is usually necessary. In the presence of aortic regurgitation, it may be possible to repair the dissection by suturing the dissected layers of proximal aorta together. If this is not successful, it may be necessary to replace the valve itself, with replacement of the aortic root and re-implantation of the coronaries.

Type B dissections are exposed through a left posterolateral thoracotomy. In all cases the groin is prepared and exposed for possible cannulation. Tube graft replacement is almost always necessary. Low-porosity materials are used. Newer fabrics such as collagen-impregnated double-velour Dacron are gaining popularity. These are softer and easy to handle. Resection of the aorta can be accomplished by simple cross-clamping, partial cardiopulmonary bypass (femorofemoral or atriofemoral), or heparin-bonded (Gott) shunts, usually aortofemoral.

Specific risks of this operation are:

- paraplegia (10%)
- acute renal failure
- chylothorax
- stroke
- perioperative myocardial infarction.

Peripheral vascular surgery in the cardiac patient

The postoperative coronary and valvular cardiac patient is prone to vascular complications, not only from his generalised arterial disease, but also because of the various procedures affecting his cardiovascular system, starting with the cannulation and cross-clamping of the aorta, prostheses and incisions in the heart, endothelial and blood trauma, and the insertion of devices inside the bloodstream, such as monitoring and investigational catheters and the intra-aortic balloon pump. Acute postoperative ischaemia of the limbs is caused by embolism (atrial fibrillation, heart valve prosthesis, ventricular thrombosis after MI, left ventricular aneurysm, endocardial resection, left atrial myxoma, bacterial endocarditis), thrombosis of a vascular graft on the aorta or femoral arteries, and haemorrhage and compression on vascular suture lines.

The typical presentation can be summarised by the 'multiple Ps':

- pain

- paralysis
- paraesthesia
- pallor
- perishing cold
- pulselessness
- putrification (in advanced cases).

Since most postoperative cases are due to embolism, the basic management is surgical, under local or general anaesthesia. The object is to remove the embolus using Fogarty catheters, with the patient heparinised. Postoperative anticoagulation is continued. As with IABP we keep the ACT around 250 by means of hourly heparin.

Vascular access

1. *Common femoral artery.* Patient supine with the knee slightly flexed and the hip externally rotated. The incision runs from the mid-inguinal point to the apex of the femoral triangle, and the deep fascia of the thigh is sectioned distal to the inguinal ligament. The superficial circumflex iliac vein is divided as it runs from lateral to medial to join the long saphenous vein. The common femoral artery is exposed.
2. *Brachial artery.* The arm is supported at 90° to the body with the hand supinated. A vertical incision is made in the middle of the cubital fossa, medial to the biceps tendon. The medial cubital vein is ligated and the bicipital aponeurosis divided. The median nerve is thereby exposed. Lateral to this, running towards the junction of the pronator teres and brachioradialis muscles, runs the brachial artery.
3. *Internal jugular vein.* Patient in Trendelenburg position. The head is rotated away from the site of access. The vein is then cannulated by perforating the skin of the neck at the lateral border of the sternomastoid muscle, two fingers above the clavicle. The needle is aimed just under the muscle, with an angle of 30° from the horizontal plane towards the nipple and advanced gently until blood is aspirated.
4. *Subclavian vein.* Patient in Trendelenburg position. The skin is perforated two fingers-breadth lateral and inferior to the junction of the medial and middle thirds of the clavicle. The needle may be advanced either to the sternal notch, scraping the undersurface of the bone until blood is aspirated, or to the middle point of the two bellies of the sternomastoid (Sedillot's point), where the internal jugular joins the subclavian vein.

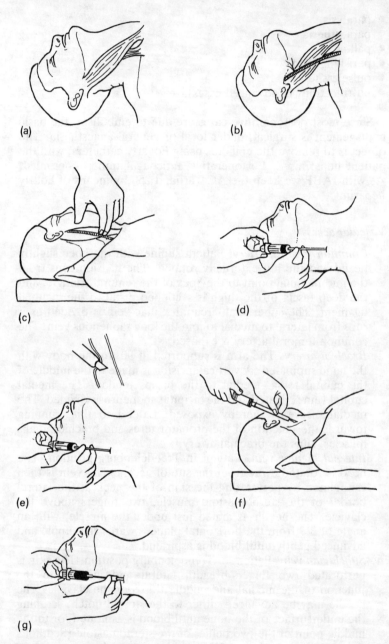

(a)

(b)

(c)

(d)

(e)

(f)

(g)

Figure 2.6 (a)–(g) Accessing the internal jugular vein

Pericardiectomy

Pericardiectomy is usually performed for constrictive pericarditis, which impairs ventricular diastolic filling. This may be due to virus, bacterial infections including tuberculosis, malignancy, collagen diseases and uraemia.

The patient usually presents with cardiac failure, predominantly right sided. The most common signs are:

- raised jugular venous pressure
- Kussmaul sign (inspiratory filling of neck veins)
- ascites
- hepatosplenomegaly
- ankle oedema
- pericardial rub
- arrhythmias (usually atrial fibrillation).

The basic investigations are:

1. Chest X-rays, which show pericardial calcification in 40% of cases.
2. Electrocardiogram, usually with low voltage and diffuse non-specific ST and T wave changes.
3. Echocardiogram, with rapid early ventricular filling.
4. Cardiac catheterisation:
   (a) equal right atrial, left atrial and pulmonary arterial pressures;
   (b) prominent x and y descents in atrial pressure;
   (c) equal LVEDP and RVEDP.

Pericardiectomy may be performed through either median sternotomy or left anterior thoractomy. This is usually difficult and may be dangerous. The parietal pericardium is removed as far back as the phrenic nerves and around the cavae as far as possible, and the epicardial calcification is removed as much as safely possible, beginning with the left ventricular surface.

Postoperatively there may be marked dilatation of the ventricles, usually the right once it is freed, leading to low cardiac output. These patients are maintained with a high left atrial pressure and inotropic support for at least 24 hours after the operation. Intra-aortic balloon pumping may be necessary.

Hospital mortality is 5–15%.

Surgery for ventricular tachyarrhythmias in ischaemic heart disease

Ventricular tachyarrhythmias complicating myocardial infarction may be divided into those of the acute phase ('early'), which occur in the first 24–48-hour period and are due to multiple transient arrhythmogenic substrates, and those occurring in a later subacute phase ('late'), which are usually due to fixed anatomical substrates.

The former are by definition self-limiting, while the latter by reason of their fixed nature are likely to be recurrent.

The late arrhythmias originate in the abnormal subendocardium and border zones of the infarcted areas and are usually re-entrant in type. Because these late arrhythmic substrates are identifiable by various pre- and intra-operative mapping techniques, they are amenable to surgical attack.

The aim of surgery is to remove or interrupt the re-entry circuit while causing minimal further impairment of ventricular function. Theoretical anti-arrhythmic surgical options include endocardial resection, encircling endocardial ventriculotomy, cryoablation or laser photocoagulation surgery. These procedures may be combined with infarctectomy or aneurysmectomy and coronary vascularisation.

The earliest site of activation in ventricular tachyarrhythmias related to infarction is located in the endocardium. To ensure the complete removal of the offending tissue it is necessary accurately to localise the arrhythmic substrates by intra-operative electrophysiological mapping. There are various types of mapping, all of them are performed on normothermic bypass:

- activation mapping in ventricular tachycardia
- fragmentation mapping in sinus rhythm
- paced mapping
- cryotermination mapping
- pressure mapping
- subthreshold stimulation mapping.

A bipolar reference electrode is sited in a normal piece of ventricular myocardium and a roving bipolar electrode used to map comprehensively first the epicardial surfaces of the right and left ventricles and later the endocardial surface of the left ventricle. In our unit a 53-point epicardial and 36-point endocardial map is constructed. The local electrogram at each point is timed relative to the reference electrode. A 200 ms delay is arbitrarily added on to the activation time so that points activated even ahead of the reference electrode will still give a positive reading.

Activation mapping is the most commonly employed intra-operative mapping technique. Sustained normomorphic ventricular tachycardia is first induced by programmed electrical stimulation. Each epicardial ventricular point is mapped and an activation time calculated. The point with the earliest activation is the epicardial breakthrough point of the tachycardia. Epicardial mapping alone is insufficient to guide surgery, as the epicardial breakthrough point may be some distance from the endocardial origin of the arrhythmia. For this reason it is necessary to open the ventricle using a ventriculotomy through the most abnormal segment and perform endocardial mapping of the left ventricle. The earliest endocardial point indicates the origin of the arrhythmia. Limitations to this technique are: arrhythmias non-inducable at operation, poorly tolerated arrhythmias which may further impair ventricular function during prolonged mapping, and unmappable arrhythmias (polymorphic VT or VF).

Fragmentation mapping is performed in sinus rhythm and is based on identifying locally abnormal points with a capacity to sustain re-entrant arrhythmias.

At the time of chest closure it is advisable to insert two atrial and two ventricular temporary electrodes for dual chamber pacing if required in the early hours postoperatively. These also facilitate diagnosis of arrhythmias in the postoperative period and the ventricular wires can be left in for electrophysiological testing prior to discharge from hospital.

As a result of the extensive surgery involved, the major problem for the patient is ventricular function in the postoperative period. The highest mortality is from cardiogenic shock and intensive support is often required in this period. Early recourse to intra-aortic balloon counterpulsation is always advisable in severe cases. The excessive use of inotropics may be counterproductive.

All patients are anticoagulated once the chest drains are removed, to reduce the chance of embolisation from thrombi forming on the roughened endocardium. This anticoagulation is continued for 3 months and then withdrawn.

At approximately 7–10 days a postoperative electrophysiological test is performed using the ventricular wires.

Acid–base balance and metabolic disturbances
Physiology
- Hydrogen ion concentration in blood may be expressed as pH or, less frequently, in nanoequivalents (nEq). pH units were

Table 2.17

pH	[H+] (nEq)
6.9	126
7.0	100
7.1	79
7.2	63
7.3	50
7.4	40
7.5	32
7.6	25

proposed by Sorensen to circumvent the difficulty of working with very low numbers.

- Acid production from metabolism in the human averages 12 000 mEq every day. Catabolism produces CO_2; metabolism of phospholipids, nucleoproteins and amino acids produce other acids.
- The main buffers in the blood are inorganic phosphates, bicarbonate, plasma proteins and haemoglobin.
- Cellular buffers: the hydrogen passing into the cells in exchange for potassium.
- Extracellular buffers, especially bicarbonate, neutralise the acids and lead to CO_2 production.
- Pulmonary compensation: increased respiratory rate and depth excrete the extra CO_2.
- Renal correction: increasing the bicarbonate production and excretion of ammonia.

Metabolic acidosis

This is caused by two mechanisms:

1. Increased acid production (abnormal cellular metabolism, ingestion of acid precursors such as methanol and salicylates).
2. Loss of bicarbonate (either by gastrointestinal diseases or by renal failure).

The early haemodynamic consequences of acidosis are increased cardiac output and lowered peripheral resistance. Late consequences are myocardial depression and increased pulmonary vascular resistance.

Metabolic acidosis may be divided according to the so-called anion gap. In normal situations, the sum of anions (Na^+, K^+, Ca^{2+}, Mg^{2+}) equals the sum of cations (Cl^-, HCO_3^-, proteins, sulphates, phosphates). The sum of $Na^+ + K^+$ represents 95% of cations of extracellular fluid, whilst the sum of $Cl^- + HCO_3^-$ accounts for 85% of extracellular anions.

In the relation
$$Na^+ + K^+ = Cl^- + HCO_3^- + X$$

X is the amount of non-measurable anions, normally around 15 mmol/litre. Therefore;

$$X = (Na^+ + K^+) - (HCO_3^- + Cl^-) = 15$$

According to this, metabolic acidosis may be classified into:

1. Acidosis with normal anion gap (gastrointestinal disease, renal disease).
2. Acidosis with high anion gap (diabetes, starvation, alcoholic intoxication, lactic acidosis, salicylates, methyl alcohol, renal failure).

General treatment

1. Investigation and treatment of the cause.
2. Intravenous sodium bicarbonate, especially if the pH falls below 7.2 and/or the serum bicarbonate goes below 12 mmol/ litre.

Note that i.v. bicarbonate may impair tissue oxygenation and also precipitate acute pulmonary oedema. It is given according to the formula:

(24 − real bicarbonate) × 50% of body weight.

The initial dose over the first hour should be one-third of the calculated total dose. The next third is given over the next 6–8 hours and the last third over the next 12 hours.

Blood gas levels are measured frequently, especially the base excess. Peritoneal dialysis and haemodialysis may become necessary. Beware of metabolic alkalosis and hypokalaemia.

Metabolic alkalosis

Metabolic alkalosis is compensated by increasing hydrogen coming from phosphates and proteins, CO_2 retention and renal excretion of bicarbonate.

Clinical signs mainly relate to associated electrolytic disturbances: hypokalaemia and hypocalcaemia.

Main causes of metabolic alkalosis are:

1. Associated with loss of extracellular volume: vomiting, gastric drainage, diuretics.
2. Associated with normal extracellular volume. Excess of mineralocorticoids: hyperaldosteronism, Cushing's syndrome, hypokalaemia.
3. Others. Exogenous administration of alkaline substances.

Treatment is aimed at correction of the underlying disease and the associated hypokalaemia.

Peri-operative infection in cardiac surgery

The host

Cardiac patients are at a higher risk of developing infections compared to other surgical patients. Contributory factors are:

- greater age
- diabetes
- obesity
- malnutrition
- renal failure
- reoperation
- cardiopulmonary bypass
- insertion of prosthetic material
- prolonged operative times
- invasive monitoring
- reduced cardiac output
- intravascular circulatory assistance
- endotracheal ventilation
- tracheostomy
- prolonged hospitalisation.

In transplanted patients immunosuppression largely increases infective risks. Timely surgery, meticulous asepsis, effective prophylaxis, and proper management in the ITU are required to minimise these hazards.

Sources

Preoperative cultures of urine, throat, nose, and perineum and antibody titres against hepatitis B and HIV are routinely done. Teeth are checked.

At operation, hands should be scrubbed for 5 minutes with any approved agent if the surgeon has not scrubbed within the past week. Between operations, shorter scrubs are advisable. If anyone has a cutaneous or upper-respiratory or viral infection, then he or she should ideally not operate, nor should anyone who is a 'carrier' of a dangerous staphylococcus.

General good theatre design, simple common sense and good surgical discipline are more important factors than sophisticated attempts actively to sterilise the environment.

Infection may occur in the ITU particularly if prolonged stay is required. Personnel in the ward should always wash their hands between examining the patients, in particular after contact with infected patients.

Preparation of the operative field

Showers with antiseptic soap start the day before operation, and chlorhexidine powder is applied to groins and axillae. Cardiac surgery usually requires extensive shaving, but shaving may predispose to wound infection, particularly if it is too early and the skin is broken. Naseptin cream is put into the nostrils.

Provided all investigations, including dental, are negative, preparation of the operative field in theatre is carried out with spirit-based povidone–iodine (1% in 70% ethyl alcohol). Once drying has occurred, effective asepsis of the skin has been achieved. (Care must be taken to avoid the streaming of iodine outside of the operative field and on sensitive areas like perineum, genitalia or face.) If a history of iodine sensitivity is present then other techniques and other antiseptic solutions with similar effectiveness can be used.

Prophylactic antibiotics in cardiac surgery

Cardiac surgery, unless an active endocarditis is present, is a clean procedure. The likeliest and the most troublesome bacteria are the staphylococci and, in particular, *Staph. aureus*. Although broad spectrum antibiotics (usually cephalosporins) have been advocated by many surgeons, narrow spectrum penicillin-derived antibiotics seem to be the most logical answer to the staphylococci. This avoids multi-resistant organisms and has minimal side-effects. We recommend flucloxacillin as the antibiotic of choice in both valve and coronary surgery. The greatest fears are mediastinitis and prosthetic valvular endocarditis (see p. 126).

Postoperative fever

1. *Pulmonary* infections are likelier with previous pulmonary vascular or airways pathology, prolonged ventilation, reoperation for bleeding, and tracheostomies. Early there may be pulmonary neutrophilic sequestration, complement activation and atelectasis. Later purulent secretions, hypoxia, atalectasis, and positive sputum-cultures (usually *H. influenzae* and *Strep. pneumoniae*) confirm the diagnosis.
2. *Vascular catheter* infections are usually staphylococci and diphtheroids.
3. *Urinary tract* infection may cause Gram-negative septicaemia.
4. *Unknown* sources underlie 30% of postoperative bacteraemia.
5. *Non-infective* fever may result from post-pericardectomy syndrome (fever, pericardial rub, leukocytosis, pleural effusion) but this must be a diagnosis of exclusion, which should include thrombophlebitis, drug reactions and pulmonary embolisation.

Median sternotomy wound infection – mediastinitis

Infections of the sternal wound are uncommon following cardiac surgery and range from minor superficial infection to sternal dehiscence and suppurative mediastinitis.

Incidence

This has been reported to be 0.8–1.5% but can be as high as 8% when bilateral internal mammary artery to coronary artery bypass grafting is performed. Recently, however, the latter has been proved to be limitable to 2.6%.

Predisposing factors

Diabetes mellitus, obesity, prolonged pre-operative hospitalisation and prolonged operative time, co-existing infection elsewhere in the body, old age, reoperation and undrained retrosternal haematoma predispose to infective wound complications. Nevertheless, imperfect aseptic technique in the operating room, as well as inaccurate and insecure sternal closure, are the basic causes of the infection.

Bacteriology

The vast majority of bacterial isolates are *Staph. aureus, Staph. albus, Staph. epidermidis* and rarely diptheroides and coliforms.

Gram-negative bacilli have been also reported to be responsible for severe forms of mediastinitis.

Clinical findings

1. Unusual fever and malaise, sternal tenderness and persistent severe central chest pain without necessarily obvious inflammation of the skin.
2. Drainage from below the sternum or accompanied by sternal instability.
3. Persistent local purulent drainage with persistent pyrexia.

Diagnosis

1. Examination.
2. Culture.
3. CT scan may identify a retrosternal abscess or sternal disruption.

Diagnosis should be made before there is extensive breakdown of the wound skin edges.

Treatment

1. *Superficial wound infection:* proper drainage and débridement. If cellulitis is present, appropriate antibiotics.
2. *Mediastinitis:* return to theatre after obtaining blood and wound cultures. The entire incision should be reopened and all foreign material (sutures, wires, pacing wires, etc.) removed. All infected and necrotic tissue should be débrided and the sternum scraped, removing minimal bone. Care should be taken to avoid entering any uninfected planes. Multiple cultures are obtained and, pending sensitivities, broad spectrum antibiotics are given and continued for ten days i.v. followed by one week orally. The wound and mediastinum are irrigated with diluted Betadine. Two small size (16–18 F) chest drains are inserted anteriorly for aspiration of diluted 0.5% Betadine or antibiotic irrigation. The sternum is closed with wires around the cortical bone, and all–layer closure done superficial to this. Betadine irrigation starts at a rate of 1–2 ml/kg/hour and continues for 6–7 days, after which time the drains become sequestrated and should be removed. A detailed record is maintained of the total infused and drained amount of fluid. Should the balance become positive by more than 100 ml,

the infusion is stopped until the fluid is recovered. A chest radiograph is required every 2–3 days to identify any fluid entering the pleural space. Cultures are obtained regularly from the drained fluid.

Open method: if infection persists then, after careful re-exploration and second débridement, the wound is left open and packed with Betadine gauze. Daily dressings are applied and the secondary closure carried out 12–15 days later. The use of pedicle flaps (both pectoralis major muscles and/or rectus abdomini) may reduce morbidity.

Continuous irrigation should be successful in 90%, but if other methods are necessary, the mortality is 20–40%. Meticulous asepsis and accurate surgical technique can keep the incidence down to 0.1%.

Sternal non-union

This occurs in patients with chronic bronchitis, emphysema, asthma or pneumonia, even in the absence of wound infection. The wires should go around the sternum rather than through it, and be at maximum tension.

Prosthetic valve endocarditis (PVE)

PVE affects 1–3% of all cardiac valves implanted; 4–5% of valve recipients, mainly during the first year after surgery. The mortality approaches 50%.

Bacteriology

- *Staph. aureus*
- *Staph. epidermidis*
- diphtheroids
- pseudomonas
- fungi
- normally-saprophytic organisms.

Contamination frequently occurs in the operating theatre.

Predisposing factors

- long operation
- prolonged stay in ITU
- low cardiac output

- bacteraemia (dental abscesses, diverticulitis, etc.)
- other cryptic infections elsewhere in the body
- male sex
- native endocarditis.

Pathology

Abscess (40–60%) may occur, usually between the sewing ring of the valve and the surrounding tissues. The suturing of the valve is threatened and, should a large abscess develop (for example, in the intraventricular septum), sudden fistula or regurgitation may occur. Formation of bulky vegetations (1.5%) may obstruct the valve.

Diagnosis

- pyrexia
- weakness
- signs of cardiac failure and persistent bacteraemia in the absence of an extrathoracic source
- prosthetic malfunction
- systemic emboli (15–20%)
- anaemia
- microscopic haematuria
- elevated sedimentation rate
- increased concentration of circulating immune complexes.

Early development (2–3 months after surgery) indicates nosocomial infection.

Investigations

1. Cultures: if PVE is suspected, multiple (> 10) blood cultures should be obtained during the first 24 hours. All potential primary sites of infection should be cultured.
2. ECG: progressive atrioventricular or bundle branch conduction disturbances.
3. Chest X-ray: signs of cardiac failure.
4. Echo and catheter: evidence of excessive mobility or dysfunction of the prosthesis.

Treatment

If cultures are positive, appropriate i.v. antibiotics; if cultures are negative, broad spectrum antibiotics – vancomycin, gentamicin and ampicillin. Antibiotics should be continued for 6–8 weeks.

Surgical intervention

Fifty per cent will require surgery to débride infection and correct haemodynamics. Although antibiotic therapy for 10 days before operation is preferable, surgery has to be carried out before haemodynamic deterioration becomes irreversible.

Indications

1. NYHA grade 3 and 4 because of SBE-induced dysfunction.
2. Evidence of invasive infection:
   (a) echocardiographic evidence of valvular dehiscence or dysfunction;
   (b) progressive electrocardiographic conduction system disturbances;
   (c) persistent unexplained pyrexia despite appropriate antimicrobiological therapy.
   (d) purulent pericarditis.
3. Fungal endocarditis.
4. Relapse of infection after adequate medical treatment.
5. Recurrent thromboembolic episodes.
6. Persistent positive blood cultures despite full antibiotic therapy.

Early PVE is more likely to require surgery, whereas after one year antibiotics alone may suffice.

Postoperative management and results

Appropriate antibiotics should be continued for a minimum of four weeks postoperatively. Anticoagulation starts the second postoperative day in patients with mechanical valves and in patients with a history of systemic emboli. Extra-cardiac infection can result in re-infection of the new prosthetic valve. Prophylactic antibiotic therapy should be administered to all patients undergoing subsequent surgical procedures.

The hospital outcome depends on the degree of pre-operative heart failure, and the type and severity of infection. The operative mortality is 15% in good centres for late PVE and as high as 50–60% for early. The recurrent infection rate is approximately 5%.

Effects of sepsis on myocardial function

Sepsis affects myocardial performance irrespective of the underlying heart disease and demands greater cardiac performance.

1. *Periphery*. There is an increased demand by the tissues, hence:
    (a) peripheral vasodilatation; selective vasoconstriction occurs in muscles, skin and abdominal organs with increased flow to brain, heart and kidneys. Later still, toxic, passive collapse of vasomotor tone occurs.
    (b) a shift of the oxyhaemoglobin dissociation curve to the right facilitates the delivery of oxygen.
2. *Cardiac function*. The determinants of cardiac output are: ventricular preload, contractility, afterload and rate.

Preload

The left ventricular preload should be expressed as an end-diastolic volume (LVEDV), but is normally estimated as the end-diastolic pressure (LVEDP), risking mistakes by ignoring the diastolic compliance of the LV (LVDC). Nevertheless, a Swan–Ganz catheter permits some assessment of the haemodynamic profile, important in septic patients.

Sepsis reduces the ventricular compliance (LVDC) and thus small volumes have an exaggerated effect on the pulmonary capillary wedge pressure (PCWP), especially in cardiac ischaemia, or patients receiving inotropic support with high LV preload to maximise output. Further increase may thus not increase the output but may exceed the peak of the ventricle's 'Starling curve'. It is better to improve the compliance and reduce the afterload; a pericardial effusion must be drained and vasodilators used. Improved LVDC allows greater LV preload expansion (by volume) and hence augmented stroke volume by the Frank–Starling mechanism.

LV contractility

Endotoxins reduce LV contractility but, in the very early stages of sepsis, contractility may be improved by circulating and endogenous catecholamines. Later the production of a lysosomal enzyme (myocardial depressing factor; MDF) in the ischaemic splanchnic region depresses LV contractility.

In chronic cardiac disease, there is reduced beta-adrenergic receptor modulation of myocardial contractility. Prolonged endogenous or therapeutic catecholamine stimulation causes myocardial damage (myofibrillar degeneration) and a down-regulation of the cardiac beta-receptors. In septic cardiac patients, this reduced beta-receptor function becomes more apparent and explains the LV contractile state in sepsis being unchanged by circulating catecholamines and decreased LV afterload.

LV afterload

The systemic peripheral vascular resistance (SPVR) is characteristically low in sepsis, which facilitates ventricular ejection and increases the CO. Later, however, with selective vasoconstriction the SPVR rises, increasing LV stroke work and, with the toxic myocardial depression, this leads to cardiac failure. A vasodilator (nitroglycerine) may thus maintain the CO, but this must be administered cautiously as diastolic blood pressure and, therefore, coronary perfusion, may fall too far.

RV afterload

In sepsis, this is raised. Pulmonary hypertension (PH), for example in chronic mitral valve stenosis, increases the mortality of sepsis. the RV is less able to increase its contractile function because of its thin wall.

The pressure gradient which determines the venous return to the right atrium (RA) is: mean systemic pressure − RA pressure. An increased RA pressure as a result of elevated RA afterload (due to increased PVR, due to sepsis) may potentially limit this. Reduction of venous compliance or volume infusion might be required.

RV preload

In sepsis the RV compliance too is reduced. The RV is very thin, especially when full, so pericardial effusions will particularly affect the preload and must be drained.

RV contractility

RV hypertrophy, as in mitral stenosis or in chronic obstructive lung disease, provides greater contractile reserve. Toxic RV contractile depression, after increasing preload as far as possible, may be helped by the infusion of pulmonary vasodilators (nitroglycerine) systemically or into the PA (prostacyclin).

RV dilatation may alter the LV geometry: left septal shift may reduce LV filling and hence CO.

Peroperative nursing care of the cardiac surgical patient

Before operation

The rôle of the nurse interested in cardiac disease must be to give emotional as well as physical support to patients and their relatives and to devise an acceptable health education programme to make life more enjoyable again.

Ideally a pre-operative programme of perhaps six weeks could help the patient to be in better control of his life, toning him up and ensuring peak fitness, both physically and mentally, for his impending surgery. He will then feel he has contributed towards his treatment for this devastating disease, and will worry less about the forthcoming operation.

The pre-operative programme should include a very gentle exercise programme; we suggest exercises as encouraged in the Health Education Council's *Look After Yourself* course, which encourages basic physical fitness, but not to athletic standards. Relaxation is an important part of life and therefore the patient should be taught basic relaxation techniques, perhaps encouraged with a relaxation tape. Education is also required in reduction of stress. During this programme, the patient is directed towards healthier diet, free of fats, sugar and salt and high in dietary fibre. Smoking should have been banned at a very early stage in the history of the patient's heart disease. If the patient is nevertheless smoking then ideally six weeks should come between stopping and surgery to decrease the chances of complications.

A psychological assessment may reveal problems which can be identified and treated prior to surgery.

This programme should be carried out with the help of the patient's relatives as it is important that they also understand the principles of the programme and the risk factors involved.

Patients for cardiac surgery should be admitted at least two days prior to surgery, but it is probable that some patients have cardiac surgery as an emergency procedure and therefore the pre-operative programme must be explained and adopted postoperatively.

On admission to a cardiac surgical ward the nurse must assess the patient and his problems must be recorded in the appropriate documents. A problem-solving approach may then be initiated and updated continuously. The nurse must instil confidence into the patient, ensuring a common goal of purpose in the nurse–patient relationship. Introduction to the ward, other patients, staff and ward routines is essential, as are reassurance and explanation of all procedures to be carried out. The nurse must also remember we are now in control of the patient's life; he has lost his normal control and can no longer dictate or control his environment.

A two-day cycling programme on an ergometric exercise bike whilst in hospital will increase the patient's confidence and his awareness of his exercise thresholds.

This period must be used to reduce the risk of infection prior to surgery. Once the patient has settled into the ward and is feeling more comfortable, he should have a Hibiscrub shower and hair wash and then put on freshly laundered pyjamas. Outside clothes should be kept in a separate locker or sent home until the patient feels well enough postoperatively to want to wear them. The patient must be encouraged to take a daily Hibiscrub shower until the day of his operation; an antibacterial powder may be used for the axilla, groins and perineal areas twice a day and an antiseptic nasal cream twice a day, to reduce aggressive skin flora.

Whilst in hospital, the patient should be encouraged to continue his relaxation exercises to prepare him psychologically for his forthcoming operation. It is important to remember that an aggressive or irritable patient is usually frightened and needs constant reassurance and explanations. Everything about his stay in hospital should be explained by the nurse, including the operation (although the doctor will have explained the procedure), his time in the intensive therapy unit and all the invasive monitoring which will be in use, his return to the ward and his subsequent rehabilitation. Talking to other patients who have had their operation and are ready for discharge should also be of great benefit to the patient and will let him see what to expect, and what is expected of him.

On the morning of operation the nurse's first priority is to reassure the patient. The relaxation techniques he has been taught will be very helpful at this stage. The patient should have a Hibiscrub shower and hair wash; the skin is prepared using an antiseptic solution, for example iodine or chlorhexidine, and the patient should then put on a theatre gown. Once in his cleanly-made bed, the premedication should be given as prescribed and the usual pre-theatre check carried out. Reassurance should be given constantly throughout this procedure, and during transfer to theatre.

The recovery phase

Following cardiac surgery the main task of the ITU is accurate and continuous monitoring of the patient's clinical and physiological condition to enable early diagnosis and prompt treatment of any complications. Every patient needs at least one experienced intensive care nurse at the bedside all the time.

Peripheral and central temperature

These are observed constantly, since they are affected early in cases of low cardiac output. Patients following cardiac surgery return to intensive care with a central temperature of 36°C. A space-blanket is used until the central temperature is normal. A pyrexia of 38°C is common on the evening following surgery and, although it rarely requires treatment, the possibility of infection should be taken into account.

Cardiac rhythm and rate

Recognition of departure from sinus rhythm and the main cardiac arrhythmias is basic, since these can be life-threatening (ventricular fibrillation), may reduce cardiac output (tachycardias, bradycardias), or may simply be the manifestation of electrolyte imbalance (ventricular ectopics).

Invasive monitoring

This technology is vital in the minute-by-minute management of the patient. The following parameters can be obtained: systolic, diastolic and mean atrial pressure; right arterial pressure; left atrial pressure; pressures obtained by pulmonary flotation catheters. Therefore, it is essential that the nurse can read the monitors. Any recording should be considered in the context of the patient's general condition (e.g. a blood pressure recording of 120/80 is not satisfactory if the patient is peripherally cold, his skin clammy and his urinary output poor).

To provide observations which are consistent requires correct positioning of the transducer in relation to the patient. The zero level of the transducer head is the mid-axillary line, level with the patient's nipple. Accuracy is ensured by using a spirit level. The level of the transducer should be altered when the position of the patient is changed. Patency of the cannula is maintained by a continuous slow flush of 3 ml/h using commercially available, disposable systems. Sodium metabisulphite is added to the 500 ml sodium chloride used to flush venous lines; this prevents contamination of the cannula tip. Sodium metabisulphite must *not* be added to the bag flushing the arterial line.

Care of the cannula site

All sites of insertion should be clean and as infection-free as possible. The external cannula should be secured in such a way that there is no kinking or displacement. Rapid blood loss can be caused by loose connections or disconnection from cannulae. The circulation distal to the arterial cannula is checked, as emboli may occur.

The right atrial and pulmonary cannulae may be used to administer inotropic support so, before injecting any bolus to check patency, a sample must be withdrawn and discarded in order to remove traces of the inotrope before flushing.

The left atrial cannula can be dangerous – its tip is in the left side of the heart. Therefore, extra care should be taken not to inject air which can go to the peripheral vessels, including the cerebral arteries. Also, removal of this line within 24 hours from surgery should be performed at least one hour prior to removing mediastinal drains, as haemorrhage may cause cardiac tamponade.

Fluid and electrolyte balance

An accurate fluid balance record ensures adequate hydration, enabling a low urinary output to be distinguished as being due to low blood volume or low cardiac output. The most common electrolyte disturbance is hypokalaemia; regular monitoring of serum K^+ levels prevent its complications, especially if the patient is having a large diuresis.

Mediastinal drains

At the end of cardiac surgery, two mediastinal drains are left in situ. They are attached to suction 30 mmHg or 4 kPa. The amount of drainage is recorded every 30 minutes and continual assessment of blood balance is thus possible.

The nurse must note drainage type, the presence of clotting in the tubes, pattern of drainage (continuous increase or abrupt cessation). The drains should be 'milked' periodically to maintain patency. When drains are removed, the nurse checks that they are complete in length.

Temporary pacing

Potential or actual heart block at surgery is managed by inserting temporary epicardial wires connected to an external pacing box.

The ability to distinguish between the various types of pacing on the ECG monitor is important:

- ventricular pacing
- atrial pacing
- AV sequential pacing
- patient's own rhythm successfully inhibiting artificial pacing.

Efficient observation will detect any failure to pace, which may be due to:

- flat batteries
- non-insulated wires touching the skin
- wires touching each other causing a short circuit
- loose connections
- broken wire
- electrode in unsatisfactory position
- threshold increased for some other reason, so that the external box provides insufficient impulse to trigger the heart.

The wires are left *in situ* until removal of sutures or longer if necessary.

Intra-aortic balloon pump

Insertion of IABP is usually in theatre but may also be performed in ITU. Percutaneous insertion is the route of choice but technical difficulties may require a surgical incision. The recognition of poor augmentation by observation of the ECG and arterial trace on the monitor will indicate the need for adjustment.

Special nursing considerations are:

1. Position of the patient to prevent kinking of the catheter and impaired augmentation.
2. Observation of limb: poor peripheral circulation and diminished or absent foot pulses.
3. Haematoma, infection and haemorrhage.
4. Knowledge of machine: alarm system and how to reset. Monitoring of helium gas cylinder and how to change.

Removal of the percutaneous IABP requires uninterrupted pressure to the femoral artery.

Ventilation

All ventilators are set up by nursing staff prior to the patient's admission to the ITU. The medical staff are responsible for the checking, prescribing, setting ventilation (i.e. minute volume, FIO_2, inspired and expired time) and ensuring the ventilator alarm is switched on.

Continuous nursing observation is necessary. The patient's skin colour is observed and chest movements and respirations are recorded. Both sides of the chest should be expanding fully and in time with the ventilator. Ventilator observations are recorded half-hourly, including minute volume, FIO_2, upper and lower airway pressures, ventilator rate and other values taken from formulae. Ventilator temperature is measured using a servopack. This should be kept at 36–36°C and should also be recorded half hourly.

Routine bypass patients who are ventilated for less than 24 hours do not require hot-water humidification. Self-humidifying filters are used on these patients. Longer ventilation should have hot-water humidification to prevent respiratory complications. We change all ventilator circuits every 24 hours.

Many emergencies occur during mechanical ventilation, among others: blocked or kinked endotracheal tube producing a rise in airway pressure; accidental disconnection from the ventilator causing a fall in airway pressure and expiratory minute volume; blocked expiratory filter causing increase in airway pressure and increased expiratory pressure. Sometimes the endotracheal tube may become kinked, compressed, bitten or dislodged, causing abnormal respiratory movements, cyanosis and haemodynamic deterioration.

There should be an extra oxygen supply at the bedside with a hand ventilation set attached, so that in the event of an emergency the patient can be disconnected from the ventilator and hand-bagged until the problem is resolved.

It is essential to have intubation equipment readily available. A pre-set trolley or box containing all necessary equipment in order is mandatory.

The requirements for endotracheal suction for patients on intermittent positive pressure ventilation (IPPV) are:

- wall suction unit with tubing attached
- supply of sterile suction catheters of correct size
- hand cleansing lotion dispenser
- foil bowl containing sterile water.

The procedure is as follows:

1. Explain procedure to patient.
2. Ensure suction unit is functioning and set to desired vacuum range.

3. Peel open outer packet of suction catheter.
4. Remove protective cover from suction control.
5. Holding funnel-end of suction catheter with outer packet connect the suction control to the catheter.
6. Cleanse hands with lotion, using 5–10 ml in the palm of hands. Rub hands back and front to dryness, place thumb and forefinger of the right hand together, pick up catheter-end of tubing with left hand.
7. Remove suction catheter from package by holding the catheter outer packet between the palm of the right hand and small finger, keeping thumb and forefinger together. Take care not to contaminate the catheter once it is removed from the packet; grasp the suction catheter approximately 15 cm from the tip between thumb and forefinger of right hand.
8. Immediately following inspiration remove the end from swivel connector with left hand, taking care not to contaminate any part which enters the airway.
9. Introduce the suction catheter via the endotracheal tube into the trachea as far as possible. Occlude the 'T' limb of the suction control with the left forefinger and withdraw the catheter gently. This should not take longer than you can hold your own breath comfortably. If ventilator alarm goes off you have taken too long.
10. Replace end into swivel connector and ensure patient is being ventilated. Observe chest wall movements. When the servo-ventilator alarm stops sounding you know that ventilation is re-established. Dispose of catheter and flush suction connecting tube with water.
11. Procedure is repeated as often as necessary to ensure trachea is free from secretions. Always use a new disposable catheter for each aspiration and recleanse hands with the lotion. Turning the patient's head well to the right encourages the catheter tip to enter the left main bronchus.

When the suction is completed, replace caps on suction control and wash hands. Following aspiration, observe patient's ventilation.

All ventilated patients require endotracheal suction. This procedure is performed 1–2-hourly or more often, depending on the amount of secretions obtained. Early detection of chest infection is essential in the intubated patient. Therefore, sputum is observed and abnormalities reported.

Each time suction is peformed we record:

• amount obtained (small, medium, large)

- colour (mucoid, purulent, blood stained)
- type of secretions (thick, thin).

Daily sputum specimens are sent for culture and sensitivity from both intubated and extubated patients.

Routine bypass patients are ventilated for approximately 12 hours. When the patient is awake and obeying verbal commands, is cardiovascularly stable and has satisfactory blood gases, he will be taken off mechanical ventilation and allowed to breathe spontaneously. The endotracheal tube remains *in situ* until normal respirations are established and the patient is maintaining good blood gases. Oxygen is given via a face mask 3–4 litres/min. If the patient has thick secretions, 40% oxygen will be given using an Inspiron and Gilston T-piece.

After extubation, oxygen therapy continues until the patient is able to maintain adequate Po_2 on room air. Patients who have respiratory problems postoperatively may be unable to breathe spontaneously via a face mask or Gilston T-piece and a slower method of weaning may be necessary. An intermittent mandatory ventilation (IMV) circuit may be added to the ventilator circuit. This will enable the patient to do some breathing himself; if he/she cannot manage, baseline ventilation will continue. As the patient's condition improves, the minute volume and respiratory frequency can be reduced gradually.

Continuous positive airway pressure (CPAP) may be indicated in some cases.

Neurological aspects

Most patients will have a morphine infusion running at 2–3 mg/h. Patients who are candidates for early extubation have their infusions reduced to 1mg/h when they are haemodynamically stable and this is continued until the patient is due to return to the ward. Additional bolus doses of morphine and sedatives (e.g. midazolam) are prescribed to be given as necessary intramuscularly following extubation.

All patients are assessed neurologically by nursing staff as soon after theatre as possible. The patient is asked to obey simple commands, i.e. opening eyes, moving both feet, gripping with both hands. Any weakness will be recorded and reported. If the patient is unable to obey commands, the nurse will note whether the patient has a cough reflex during suction and if he grimaces during procedures which are painful or unpleasant.

Patients who are thought to have a neurological problem will have observations recorded on a Glasgow coma scale chart.

Further sedation will be avoided if possible and a neurological opinion will be sought when the patient has been without sedation long enough to be fully assessed.

Physiotherapy

Every patient should be seen by the physiotherapist pre-operatively. This helps to gain the patient's confidence and enables him to receive a clear explanation of what is expected of him postoperatively. Patients are taught diaphragmatic, lateral, costal and apical breathing. They are also told of the importance of clearing secretions, coughing and cough holds.

Reassurance is given to the patients that moving, breathing and coughing will not harm the operation site or drainage tubes. Foot and leg exercises are also taught.

The main aims are to:

1. Expand lung tissue by maximum inspiratory effort.
2. Prevent lung collapse and/or consolidation by localised breathing exercises, diaphragmatic breathing, vibration, shaking, percussion and coughing.
3. Remove excess secretions.
4. Prevent circulatory complications by foot and leg exercises, general movements and deep breathing that aids venous return.
5. Maintain joint mobility and muscle strength by exercises.
6. Maintain good posture.

If the X-ray is clear and air-entry is satisfactory it is not necessary to turn the patient from side to side during physiotherapy. Incentive spirometry is now frequently used in ITU to encourage deep breathing and prevent retention of secretion. Bird-type ventilators are also used by the physiotherapist on patients with areas of basal collapse. In an effort to loosen thick secretions prior to the physiotherapist's visit, nursing staff may be requested to give menthol inhalations to the patient. This visit should be done at least four times daily.

Skin and personal care

In the immediate postoperative phase the patient is totally dependent on the nurse for his personal hygiene. Bed-bathing should cause minimum discomfort. Any pain or anxiety which may be experienced can be alleviated by the use of analgesia and sedation. Explanation of planned movements is necessary especially if the patient has had muscle relaxants. Care should be taken not to decannulate the patient accidentally.

The blink-reflex loss from neuromuscular blocking drugs or coma may cause damage to the cornea. Prevention is by irrigating the eyes with normal saline and hypromellose eyedrops, and taping eyes closed. Eye pads of any type should be used with caution as the eyelids may open under the pads, causing corneal scratches. A swab for culture and sensitivity should be taken at any sign of infection so that the appropriate antibiotics can be administered.

The uncomplicated cardiac surgical patient is seldom at risk from pressure sores. Frequent changing of position is sufficient. Nevertheless, in cases of prolonged immobilisation for any complications, the patient might need to be nursed with the aid of a Clinitron mattress, low-air-loss bed or other pressure-relief aids. The skin must be kept dry and clean. An adequate calorie intake, especially in the debilitated patient, can reduce the severity of any problems with pressure sores and aid the healing process.

The mediastinotomy incision may be undressed the following day and sprayed with a plaster dressing. The more critically-ill patient who has a tracheostomy or a cricothyroidostomy (mini-tracheostomy) should have the wound covered until it is healed.

Pyrexia, raised white blood count, discomfort and discharge, or signs of inflammation indicate the need for culture of wound secretions.

Nutrition

On return from theatre all patients have, for intravenous maintenance therapy, either dextrose 5% or dextrose–saline with added potassium.

Patients who are extubated soon after theatre will commence oral fluids once they are stable, and will return to a low fat, low salt diet 24 hours after operation. The maintenance intravenous therapy will be reduced accordingly.

Patients staying in the intensive care unit for longer than 24 hours may require nasogastric feeding or total parenteral nutrition. If bowel sounds are present, a fine-bore nasogastric tube is passed and, after X-rays to check the position of the tube, half-strength feeds are commenced at 20–30 ml/h. The nasogastric tube is aspirated 6-hourly. If the feeds are tolerated they are changed to full strength, usually after 18–24 hours, and the rate is increased. The intravenous maintenance fluids are reduced according to how much enteral feed is tolerated.

If no bowel sounds are present, or if the circumstances indicate, total parenteral nutrition is given.

Family support and pastoral care

For obvious reasons, the patient's communication with the family is difficult, if not impossible, for the first hours after operation. Therefore the relatives should be made to feel welcome by the nursing and medical staff. Correct information which can be understood by the lay person should be given and the opportunity to ask questions permitted.

It is important to ensure that the patient's religious practices are observed and the services of the chaplain, vicar, priest, rabbi, etc. made available to the family.

Nursing care of the cardiac surgical patient in the acute post-intensive care ward

Analgesia

The patient is transferred from ITU to the acute postoperative ward the day after the operation, once he is off the ventilator and inotropes.

Sometimes the patient is still very drowsy, or feeling euphoric because he has survived the operation and returned to the ward, and so has a pain threshold higher than usual during the first few hours. However, analgesia is still a very important part of the recovery and must be given as frequently as necessary.

Fluids

Intravenous fluids should be continued until the patient is drinking properly.

Monitoring

A cardiac monitor is ordered if any dysrhythmias have been evident in ITU, but this should be removed as soon as it is no longer necessary as it may be a major cause of anxiety to the patient. Dysrhythmias may follow cardiac surgery and the nurse must record the patient's apex and pulse, reporting any abnormalities. If treatment is instituted, its progress is recorded step by step.

Mediastinal drains may have been left *in situ* if the drainage has exceeded 10 ml/hour. These drains should be milked hourly and the drainage recorded. If this increases, the surgeon must be informed. If it is less than 10 ml/h they can be removed.

A pacing box may also be connected and the nurse's responsibility is to ensure the wires to it are not crossed or touching, and to note changes in pacing response.

Observations are recorded two-hourly overnight and any major changes reported. The following morning, observations may be reduced to four-hourly if the patient has remained well.

Anti-embolic procedures

The leg wounds of patients who have had coronary artery vein grafts are redressed on the first postoperative day. The wool and crepe bandage and the dressings should be removed and any areas which are oozing should be cleaned and covered with Melolin and sealed in Opsite. This makes the dressing waterproof and therefore the patient can shower daily without the dressing becoming wet. An anti-embolic stocking can then be applied to support the donor leg and is worn constantly for the first seven days postoperatively, removed only for dressings and showers.

Elevating the legs whilst sitting down in a chair will aid drainage but calf pressure must be reduced as much as possible so, if not actively walking and using the calf muscles, the patient should recline on his bed rather than in a chair.

Mobilisation and exercise

Early mobilisation is essential following open heart surgery and this must be explained to the patient before it begins, giving him guidelines to the expected progress and overcoming any hurdles he may envisage. The patient will be encouraged to sit out of bed and, if well enough, to walk to the toilet on the first postoperative afternoon. The second day he can walk around his bed area, to the shower, toilet and, hopefully, to the dayroom for meals.

Hourly walks in the corridor should commence on the third day, initially under supervision, and the patient should be encouraged to rest, preferably on his bed, following each walk.

Mounting stairs should begin with one flight slowly at the patient's own pace, on the fourth postoperative day, increasing one flight each day to a maximum of three flights daily until the patient wishes to do more.

The postoperative cycling programme may be commenced on the fifth postoperative day and this should begin with five minutes on an ergometry exercise cycle with no resistance, and should continue twice daily until the patient feels it can be increased – a small resistance may be commenced and increased as necessary.

Each patient should have at least one hour's sleep during the day and staff should ensure this.

Older patients may have particular problems (arthritis, peripheral vascular disease, maturity onset diabetes, urological problems, etc.) which must be taken into consideration before starting a rehabiliation programme.

Physiotherapy

The patient is seen pre-operatively by the physiotherapist and deep breathing exercises, etc. are explained and the patient is taught how to breathe using the diaphragm. The physiotherapist will see the patient in the intensive care area and follow-up care will continue on the ward. The nurse is the person who is at the bedside 24 hours a day and she is the person who will encourage the patient to continue with his deep breathing exercises most of the time. The nurse must also observe the patient, his expectoration, and the amount, colour and consistency of the sputum he is expectorating. Menthol inhalations given 4-hourly will aid expectoration of secretions, provided the nurse ensures the patient uses them properly. Postural drainage is also helpful and should be encouraged whenever the patient is on his bed.

Coughing is very painful for the patient with a sternotomy and, when possible, analgesia should be given prior to any intensive physiotherapy. The patient should also be taught to support his chest when coughing; holding a pillow firmly over the sternal wound does help.

A Triflow inspirator encourages greater inspiration and deep breathing and therefore makes expectoration easier. It is also fun for the patient to use and the competitive patients on the ward will try to beat each other and some even try to cheat!

Wound care

Surgical wounds are one of the most important parts of nursing care on any surgical ward. Patients worry about their wounds from their first conscious moment after the operation. Their body image is altered and they feel insecure within their own physical dimensions.

Scrupulous asepsis must be maintained at all times during wound care. Any wound which is oozing or looking suspicious must be swabbed for culture and sensitivity. Breathing is painful and the patient feels his wound will open with each breath. Coughing, laughing and particularly sneezing can be excruciatingly painful and reassurance is needed constantly so the patient understands his capabilities.

Most wounds heal with minimal problems but some do not. The most common problems are:

1. Overdiathermy of wound edges, causing necrosis and persistent haemoserous ooze. Hydrogen peroxide will remove the necrosed tissue and enable granulation to proceed.
2. Pockets of serous fluid or blood, or skin sinuses. They may be packed with Milton and liquid paraffin or a similar solution on ribbon gauze. However, a sloughy or dirty sinus needs to be packed with a solution like chlorasol or eusol on ribbon gauze; hydrogen peroxide may be used on stubborn slough.
3. Infection, which is treated with antibiotics and local solutions like Betadine as necessary.

Daily hygiene

The patient should be encouraged to shower daily, initially with the assistance of a nurse. Profuse perspiration is common in the postoperative period.

Pyrexia

Pyrexia is common in most patients for 72 hours following surgery, usually for reasons not requiring specific treatment. Nevertheless, any high temperature must be properly investigated, especially in patients after valve surgery.

Weight

Fluid retention can be easily monitored if the patient is weighed daily before breakfast. Up to 2–3 kg overweight is usually expected after cardiac surgery. Ankle oedema will occur in most patients who are sitting in a chair for long periods. These patients should be encouraged to walk on their tiptoes for five minutes every hour to maximise the use of their calf muscles and therefore to increase venous return.

Gastrointestinal complaints

The main complaint from patients following cardiac surgery is and unpleasant taste causing nausea and anorexia. Fluids need to be encouraged, at least 80–100 ml/h, along with frequent tooth-brushing and a return to normal eating habits as soon as possible.

Nausea and vomiting need to be treated with an anti-emetic, preferably a gastric-emptying agent like metoclopramide.

Bowel habits are usually disturbed and straining must be minimised. A high fibre diet will help once the patient is eating properly but a laxative will ease the situation initially if constipation is a problem. It may be necessary to give suppositories to begin effective peristalsis.

Pressure area care

Thanks to early mobilisation, pressure sores are not usually a problem. The sacral area should be kept clean; washing with soap and water, then a light application of talcum powder should be all that is necessary.

Special situations (i.e. paraplegia) make special demands on nursing care.

Sleeping

Younger patients usually sleep with the aid of analgesics and relaxation. Older patients may need sleeping tablets as well. Posture is important and most patients need to be taught how to find a comfortable position to aid sleep.

Depression

All patients are likely to have a 'blues day', usually the second postoperative day. They wake up feeling very stiff, sore, confused, nauseated and generally unwell, which contrasts with the previous euphoric day. Dizziness, headaches, weakness and emotional weepiness are common when the patient has a bad day.

The nurse must be supportive and reassure the patient that this is normal; the patient should be allowed to express his fears and feelings, and even cry, without feeling humiliated or degraded. The nurse must be looking constantly for signs of depression in all her patients.

Peripheral nerve problems

Ulnar nerve palsy and, less commonly, radial nerve involvement, occasionally occur after median sternotomy. These problems usually settle spontaneously over the next weeks. Nevertheless, when the picture is too severe, the neurologist's opinion is sought by the medical staff.

Reassurance

Reassuring the patient is a job the nurse can do without realising it. Her presence, manner, efficiency, smile or tone of voice are all a patient needs to feel more relaxed and less worried. It is usually the nurse who is close at hand to answer those worrying questions.

Knowledge is essential in nursing and the nurse must seek it diligently but be ready to admit if she does not know the answer to a patient's question and to find someone who can answer it.

Paediatric cardiac disease

Introduction and neonatal collapse

The outstanding recent advances in the management of children with congenital heart disease have resulted from an integrated approach by paediatric cardiologists, surgeons and anaesthetists. The progress in each speciality has stimulated the others.

Cardiological investigation is now much safer and more accurate. Developments in surgery and anaesthesia have gone hand in hand. The progress is not slowing and it is exciting to contemplate the next ten years when one looks back to see what has been achieved in the past ten years.

There is a roughly inverse relationship between the incidence of various types of congenital heart disease and their complexity. The commonest lesions (such as bicuspid aortic valve, mild pulmonary valvar stenosis and small ventricular septal defect) are generally managed conservatively and have no impact on intensive care. Many common significant lesions (such as ventricular septal defect, atrial septal defect, and patent arterial duct) can be dealt with relatively easily. The rarer and more complex lesions consume a disproportionate amount of time, effort and finance.

The key to correct management is precise diagnosis. The number of ways in which congenital heart disease may be present is fairly limited, with the mode of presentation indicating the differential diagnosis. Obviously each lesion has a spectrum of severity and this will also determine the mode and the time of presentation.

Many forms of congenital heart disease present in infancy and most neonates present as emergencies. Because of this it is important for those working in intensive care to be conversant with the differential diagnosis of each mode of presentation and the initial management plan for each lesion. This section will briefly consider the differential diagnosis of neonates presenting with heart failure, neonates presenting with cyanosis, heart failure in infancy and other abnormalities.

147

Paediatric cardiac arrest

This should be distinguished from respiratory arrest. *Primary* is a defect in the heart itself; *secondary* indicates defects elsewhere causing normal hearts to stop. (Commoner – hypoxia or hypovolaemia, septicaemia, metabolic upsets and malignant disease.)

Diagnosis: unresponsive; pulseless, pale, apnoeic, dilated pupils, flat monitor.

ABCs of treatment

First stage

A – Airway Respiratory efforts but no gas moving. In small babies listen with a stethoscope over the nose. Clear the airway with fingers or wide bore sucker. Insert oropharyngeal airway (size 0 for infants, size 1 for 1 – 10 years and size 2 for older).

B – Breathing If apnoeic, clear and establish the airway and artificially ventilate with oxygen through a bag and mask of appropriate size, properly applied, moving the chest sufficiently.

C – Circulation If despite adequate ventilation circulation has not returned, apply chest compressions to the middle of the lower sternum. In babies the tips of two fingers are used, or the whole chest is encircled with both hands and the thumbs used to depress the sternum. In larger children the heel of the hand is used. The sternum should be depressed to about 20% of the anterior-posterior diameter of the chest. The compressions should last only half of the cycle to allow the heart to fill. The rate should be 120 per minute in small babies and 100 in larger children inflating the lungs every 5th beat.

Second stage
(When more help and equipment arrive)

A – Airway Substitute endotracheal intubation if continued ventilation is necessary, a mask is inadequate and time and skills permit it.

B – Breathing As above.

C – Circulation As above.

D – Defibrillation   Monitor ECG as soon as possible. In children ventricular fibrillation is less common than in adults, but DC defibrillation is as urgent. 4.5 cm paddles are used up to about 18 months, 8 cm after that, one just below the right clavicle and the other in the left mid-clavicular line at the level of the xiphisternum. Conducting cream must not bridge between the paddles. Start with 2 J/kg body weight, increasing to 3 or 4 J/kg, hyperventilate and try again, then give lignocaine (1 – 2 mg/kg i.v.) and try again. If the previous measures fail adrenaline (10 μg/kg/i.v.) bretylium (5–10 mg/kg/i.v.) and sodium bicarbonate (1 ml/kg/8.4% solution) can also be used.

E – ECG   The most common arrhythmia of children is bradycardia leading to asystole, caused by hypoxia and requiring oxygen and ventilation. Bradycardia that persists can be treated with atropine (20 μg/kg/i.v.). The only drugs that have been shown to be effective in reversing asystole are alpha-agonists like methoxamine (100 μg/kg) and alpha and beta-agonists like adrenaline. If available, pacing should be considered.

F – Fluids   Correct hypovolaemia or acidaemia. In an ITU intravenous access is usually available but the site should be checked before irritant drugs or fluids are injected. During resuscitation central lines deliver drugs more effectively than peripheral ones. Starting an infusion in a small, fat, collapsed baby can be very difficult.

Circulating volume can be replaced with 4.5% human albumin; starting with 10 ml/kg. Correct acidaemia later with arterial acid–base guidance.

Some drugs can be given via the trachea at twice the intravenous dose, diluted to 2 ml with normal saline, injected down the endotracheal tube through a feeding catheter. A large inspiration straight after injection helps absorption, but only small amounts of non-irritant drugs, and not albumen or sodium bicarbonate, can be given in this way.

Third stage
After 'successful' resuscitation the state varies from complete recovery to multisystem failure.

A/B – Airway/breathing   A more permanent nasal tube may be necessary, with sedation, muscle relaxation and mechanical ventilation and moderate hyperventilation ($Paco_2$ 3.5–4.0 kPa). Signs of aspiration, confirmed by X-ray, indicate appropriate antibiotics.

C – Circulation   The best possible cardiac output is achieved by manipulation of the heart's pre- and afterload and by increasing the myocardial contractility with inotropes. Use a central catheter for inotropes.

D – Damage limitation   Damage of the brain from hypoxia and ischaemia may provoke secondary damage when the brain swells inside the skull and compromises its blood supply. Oxygenation and ventilation help to preserve the brain, and hypertension, hyperglycaemia and hyperpyrexia must be avoided.

E – Epiphenomenon   This is caused by the arrest itself, (e.g. the aspiration of gastric contents), or produced by resuscitation – glottic and subglottic damage from intubation, oesophageal tear from oesophageal intubation, rib and sternal fractures and ruptures of liver and stomach from chest compressions, a haemopericardium from intracardiac injections, and a pneumo-thorax from using too large a tidal volume.

Results

Survival from 'true' cardiac arrests is initially about a third of all attempted resuscitations, but this falls to less than 10% for long-term survival. The long-term survival after respiratory arrest is much better at about 75%. Important features for survival are ventricular fibrillation rather than asystole, a short interval between the arrest and the resuscitation starting and a rapid response to resuscitation.

Conclusions

Although the outcome from asystole is poor, ventricular fibrillation has a reasonable prognosis if treated promptly. The best results of all are from treating respiratory arrests which would have gone on to become cardiac arrests.

Neonatal heart failure or collapse

Both presentations are usually preceded by only a short, non-specific history, such as poor feeding, irritability, lethargy and sweating. Each baby presenting in this way should undergo full examination, but attention should be concentrated particularly on the presence and character of pulses, signs of heart failure (hepatomegaly, tachypnoea, etc.) and the presence of cardiac murmurs. Investigation these days is almost entirely non-invasive.

This heading obviously covers a spectrum from those who are mildly breathless at rest to those presenting with cardiogenic shock, and initial management will be graded accordingly. Sick neonates require rapid immediate assessment and may need to be resuscitated before detailed investigations are performed. Although full investigation takes second place to resuscitation it is often appropriate to perform a quick echocardiogram to exclude hypoplastic left heart syndrome before aggressive and extensive campaigns of management are initiated. When a treatable lesion is confirmed, the infant is probably ventilated immediately and attention should be paid to early correction of acidosis and hypoglycaemia.

The differential diagnosis of cardiogenic shock includes septicaemia and metabolic abnormalities. Whilst the coexistence of beta streptococcal septicaemia with one of the abnormalities mentioned below is unlikely, it may be appropriate to cover the possibility with intravenous penicillin after blood cultures have been taken. Further resuscitation depends on the precise diagnosis but may include plasma infusion, inotropic drugs and prostaglandin infusion. Complications of heart failure or collapse will need to be dealt with individually; these may include renal failure, necrotising enterocolitis, fits, pulmonary problems and clotting abnormalities including disseminated intravascular coagulation.

Coarctation of the aorta

This is the commonest cause of heart failure or collapse in the neonate. In approximately 50% of cases there will be associated abnormalities such as ventricular septal defect, aortic valvular stenosis, mitral valve abnormalities, or more complex cardiac lesions. The cardinal physical sign is the absence of femoral artery pulses. Very sick infants may have no palpable arm pulses either, until after resuscitation. The chest X-ray is generally unhelpful, in that any abnormalities will be determined more by coexisting lesions. The ECG usually shows right ventricular hypertrophy. Echocardiography has had a profound impact in diagnosing coarctation and associated lesions. Management involves early primary repair of the coarctation (usually either an end-to-end anastomosis or a subclavian flap repair) together with, where appropriate, pulmonary artery banding, duct ligation, etc. A prostaglandin infusion is often given until the time of operation.

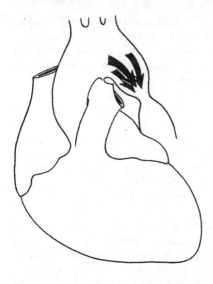

Figure 3.1 Coarctation

Hypoplastic left heart syndrome

This syndrome encompasses aortic atresia and some forms of mitral atresia. Either valve, or sometimes both, is imperforate and the left ventricle is usually very small and fibrotic. Prolonged survival is impossible and in most centres in the UK no surgical treatment is available for this condition. Once the diagnosis is established, no stabilisation or resuscitation is employed.

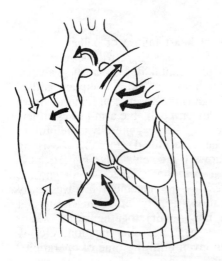

Figure 3.2 Hypoplastic left heart

These babies usually present early with tachypnoea and cyanosis, poor or absent pulses, and often marked hepatomegaly. The chest X-ray and ECG are often non-specific. The diagnosis is established by cross-sectional echocardiography; cardiac catheterisation is no longer necessary. In a few centres, experimental palliative surgery on cardiopulmonary bypass is undertaken with a view to later heart transplantation or atriopulmonary bypass. These centres will have their own protocols for management of hypoplastic left heart syndrome.

Aortic valve stenosis

The presentation of this condition in the neonate is similar to the two conditions above, from which it must be distinguished. The aortic valve is usually small and dysplastic and is often bicuspid or even monocuspid. The left ventricle may be small and dyskinetic and at the severe end of the spectrum, this condition merges with the hypoplastic left heart syndrome. As well as poor pulses there is usually an aortic ejection murmur, although this may be absent if the cardiac output is very low. After resuscitation, an aortic valvotomy is necessary in symptomatic patients. This can be achieved surgically or by transarterial balloon dilatation. With either technique the outcome is better in larger babies with less dysplastic valves but early management is still only palliative. Aortic valve stenosis may be associated with coarctation of the aorta and mitral valve abnormalities.

Supraventricular tachycardia

Surprisingly this condition is often not recognised as the baby's primary problem, despite the presence of heart failure and the heart rate of around 300/min. The maximum rate of sinus tachycardia in a sick neonate is around 220/min. The only physical signs in SVT are usually signs of heart failure and the high heart rate. The ECG shows a regular narrow QRS tachycardia at around 300/min. The substrate for the tachycardia is usually an accessory pathway and the long-term prognosis is good. The first priority is restoration of sinus rhythm. This is most easily achieved by application of an icepack to the face or facial immersion in ice-cold water. If this is ineffective, alternatives are DC cardioversion or intravenous adenosine (where available). Cardioversion is not easily repeated and requires anaesthesia. The dose of adenosine is 50 μg/kg increasing by 50 μg/kg/dose to 250 μg/kg depending on response. Intravenous verapamil is not used in neonates and infants. Once sinus rhythm is restored, maintenance anti-arrhythmic treatment is often employed for the first 6 or 12 months. Digoxin alone is often effective and, if not, the substitution of flecainide will usually maintain sinus rhythm.

Complete heart block

Even in these days of fetal ultrasound, this diagnosis is often not made *in utero* and babies are born by emergency section for presumed fetal distress. Many will not be in heart failure but symptoms develop if the ventricular rate is below 50/min. The chest X-ray may show cardiomegaly. The ECG will show a normal atrial rate with slow dissociated QRS complexes. The QRS is usually narrow. Echocardiography will identify any associated structural heart disease such as corrected transposition of the great arteries or more complex abnormalities. Permanent pacemaker implantation is indicated in those with heart failure and when the heart rate is consistently below 55/min.

In the absence of any associated structural lesion, the plasma of the mothers of most affected babies will contain anti-Ro antibodies and some will have clinical evidence of systemic lupus erythematosus or other connective tissue disease.

Transient myocardial ischaemia

This is a type of non-structural heart disease and is becoming much less common with improvements in obstetric practice. It is generally a diagnosis of exclusion. The electrocardiogram may show a variety of ST segment and T wave changes. The echocardiography may show ventricular impairment and mitral or tricuspid valve regurgitation but will exclude structural abnormalities. Treatment is supportive with dopamine infusion and correction of metabolic abnormalities, together with appropriate treatment for other ischaemic organs.

Complete atrioventricular septal defect

This is a rare presentation of this abnormality and is generally related to severe atrioventricular valve regurgitation with very dysplastic valves. The outlook is very poor and although surgical treatment may be undertaken it is rarely effective.

Patent ductus arteriosus

The duct is probably patent in almost all premature babies before 33–35 weeks gestation and closes uneventfully in the majority. A clinically significant duct most often presents in those with respiratory distress syndrome, often as they are recovering. Suspicion should be raised by tachypnoea or apnoea with an increasing $Paco_2$ on blood gases and increasing oxygen requirements. Physical examination will reveal collapsing pulses and a murmur which is more often systolic than continuous. The chest X-ray usually shows cardiomegaly, perhaps with pulmonary oedema or plethora, but interpretation may be difficult in view of the underlying lung disease. Echocardiography will demonstrate a structurally normal heart with left atrial and left ventricular volume overload. The duct can often be imaged directly but, if not, Doppler echocardiography would demonstrate the left-to-right shunt.

Initial management involves moderate fluid restriction (although this may temporarily reduce the calorie input) and a diuretic. Digoxin is often given but may not influence the course of the problem. If symptoms and signs continue and further treatment is necessary, consider indomethacin. The dose is 200 µg/kg given three times over 24 hours. It is most effective in babies of 29–33 weeks gestation and when treatment is started within 7–10 days of birth. It is most unlikely to help before 28 weeks or after 35 weeks gestation and after 3 weeks of age. Babies who fail to respond to indomethacin or are unsuitable usually require surgical ligation of the duct.

Conditions presenting with neonatal cyanosis

Neonatal cyanosis

Almost all neonates with cyanosis have either cardiac disease or pulmonary disease. A pulmonary problem is suggested by the history, by tachypnoea, by abnormal lung fields on chest X-ray and a raised $Paco_2$. If there is doubt a hyperoxia test is performed. After giving 100% oxygen to breathe for 15 minutes a right radial or brachial arterial blood gas (preductal) is taken. A $Paco_2$ higher than 30 kPa excludes cyanotic heart disease. A $Paco_2$ less than 20 kPa strongly supports cyanotic heart disease unless there is very severe lung disease. Most neonates with cyanotic heart disease require urgent assessment and treatment as they are unlikely to improve spontaneously.

Transposition of the great arteries

This is the commonest type of cyanotic heart disease in the newborn. It often presents within the first day or two and usually

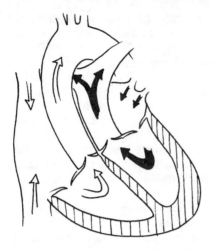

Figure 3.3 Transposition of the great arteries

within a week. If there is no VSD, physical examination is otherwise normal. The chest X-ray may show a narrow upper mediastinum but is often unhelpful except that it does not show evidence of other lesions below. The ECG is usually normal. The diagnosis is made by echocardiography which shows the pulmonary artery arising from the left ventricle and the aorta from the right ventricle. It also allows identification of associated abnormalities such as ventricular septal defect, pulmonary stenosis, etc. Initial management involves a balloon atrial septostomy. If this cannot be performed immediately an infusion of prostaglandin is given (see below) and acidosis is corrected as necessary. Further management depends on the Unit policy but involves either an atrial redirection (Mustard or Senning operation) between 6 and 12 months of life or an arterial switch within the first two weeks.

Pulmonary atresia with intact ventricular septum

In this condition the right heart is hypoplastic with an atretic right ventricular outflow, a tiny right ventricular cavity, and a very small tricuspid valve. The pulmonary arteries are usually well developed and supplied by a large duct. Clinical examination will reveal a single second heart sound and often a ductal murmur. The chest X-ray shows oligaemic lung fields, usually a normal heart size and often a concave left heart border. The ECG may show right atrial hypertrophy and sometimes left ventricular dominance. The diagnosis is established by echocardiography and particular

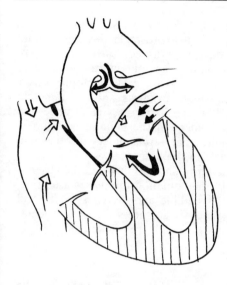

Figure 3.4 Pulmonary atresia with intact ventricular septum

attention is paid to assessment of the size and morphology of the right ventricle. Occasionally the right ventricle is well enough developed to consider a pulmonary valvotomy but early management is usually an aortopulmonary shunt. Until this is performed give a prostaglandin infusion (see below). The long-term prognosis of pulmonary atresia with intact ventricular septum is not good. The aim is to perform a right atrial–pulmonary artery anastomosis (Fontan operation or variant) in childhood but many children will not be suitable.

Pulmonary atresia with ventricular septal defect

This more commonly presents later in infancy. The ventricular anatomy is similar to that in tetralogy of Fallot, with aortic override and a large VSD. However, there is no connection between the pulmonary artery and the right ventricle. The pulmonary arterial anatomy is very variable and the true pulmonary arteries are often poorly developed. Pulmonary arterial supply is also variable, sometimes entirely via a duct and in other cases there is no duct and supply is via aortopulmonary collateral arteries. Clinical presentation and physical examination is similar to pulmonary atresia with intact septum described above. The echocardiogram will prove the diagnosis: with increasing resolution and with colour Doppler the pulmonary arterial anatomy can be defined more confidently but cardiac catheterisation is still sometimes required. Neonatal presentation suggests that the condition is duct dependent so prostaglandin is given until the presence or absence of a duct is confirmed. Early management may be conservative if the situation is stable and the pulmonary supply is not duct dependent. Otherwise early aortopulmonary shunting is performed to alleviate cyanosis and to stimulate pulmonary arterial growth. Long-term progress is variable and depends mainly on the development of the pulmonary arteries. The ideal is to close the ventricular septal defect and insert a conduit from the right ventricle to the pulmonary arteries.

This condition may present with failure to thrive in the absence of cyanosis during infancy. In that situation the pulses are brisk, continuous murmurs are easily audible and the chest X-ray will show pulmonary plethora. The ECG shows right ventricular hypertrophy.

Tetralogy of Fallot

This usually presents later in infancy or early childhood but may be detected in the newborn either if the right ventricular outflow obstruction is severe, causing cyanosis, or if a murmur is noted. Apart from cyanosis, the main physical sign is a pulmonary ejection murmur, usually with a single second sound and no ejection click. The ECG will show right ventricular hypertrophy. The chest X-ray shows a 'boot-shaped' heart with pulmonary oligaemia. The diagnosis is confirmed on echocardiography. If there is doubt about the pulmonary arterial anatomy, cardiac

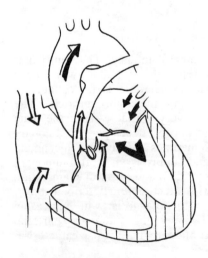

Figure 3.5 Tetralogy of Fallot

catheterisation may be required. Early management will often involve an aortopulmonary shunt. Some neonates improve spontaneously as the haemoglobin and pulmonary arterial resistance fall and a few may respond to oral propranolol. The possibility of later corrective surgery depends mainly upon the development of the pulmonary arteries.

Tricuspid atresia

The presentation depends mainly on the pulmonary blood flow. If it is diminished, cyanosis is apparent early. If it is increased, the baby will fail to thrive in early infancy and is often acyanotic. The ventricular anatomy, ventriculo-arterial connection and pulmonary arterial development are variable. The diagnosis is suspected mainly from the ECG which shows left axis deviation and left ventricular dominance. The heart's contour on chest X-ray is often 'square' but the heart size and pulmonary vascularity are variable.

In the commonest type of tricuspid atresia there is ventriculo-arterial concordance with a small ventricular septal defect producing a low pulmonary blood flow. If the foramen ovale is restrictive, a balloon atrial septostomy is performed. Prostaglandin may be given to maintain ductal patency until an aortopulmonary shunt is performed. In infants presenting with acyanotic failure to thrive, pulmonary arterial banding may be required.

Long-term prognosis is not good. A Fontan operation (right atrial–pulmonary artery connection) is the definitive repair but can only be performed if there is good pulmonary arterial

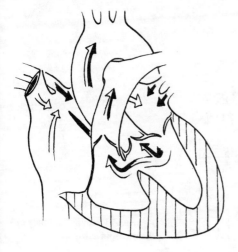

Figure 3.6 Tricuspid atresia

development, low pulmonary resistance, no distortion of the pulmonary arteries and good left ventricular function.

Ebstein's anomaly of the tricuspid valve

In this condition the tricuspid valve is dysplastic and displaced downwards into the right ventricle. The presentation depends upon the severity of the valve abnormality. Neonatal presentation implies a significantly abnormal valve and takes two main forms. If the chest X-ray shows massive cardiomegaly there is usually associated pulmonary atresia with poor pulmonary arterial development. Aortopulmonary shunting may be performed but the prognosis is usually poor. Milder forms may also present in infancy. The chest X-ray then shows a normal or slightly increased heart size. The echocardiogram confirms the diagnosis and will show tricuspid valvular regurgitation. Prostaglandin infusion is given and the baby is nursed in oxygen to encourage a rapid fall in pulmonary resistance. This will lower the right ventricular pressure, reduce the tricuspid regurgitation and thus reduce the right-to-left atrial shunting and lessen the cyanosis. Long-term prognosis can be very good. Sometimes there are associated arrhythmias (Wolff–Parkinson–White syndrome). Late cardiomegaly related to tricuspid regurgitation may necessitate tricuspid valve replacement.

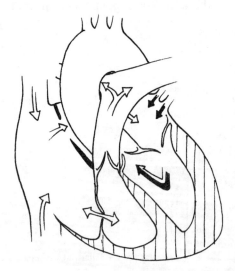

Figure 3.7 Ebstein's anomaly of the tricuspid valve

Total anomalous pulmonary venous connection

Surprisingly, presentation is often delayed for a week or two. There are usually signs of heart failure as well as cyanosis. The baby is thin, tachypnoeic and usually cyanosed. The pulmonary second sound is loud and there may be a pulmonary ejection murmur. Hepatomegaly is usual. The chest X-ray shows a small heart with pulmonary oedema. The ECG may show right ventricular hypertrophy. The diagnosis is confirmed by echocardiography which will reveal the pulmonary venous connection. With neonatal presentation the connection is often infradiaphragmatic and is usually obstructed.

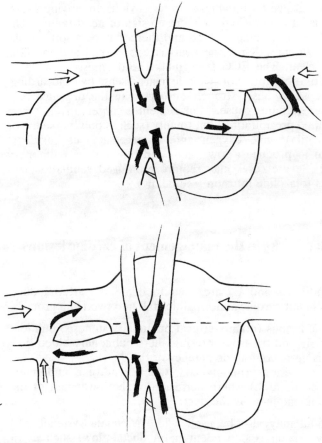

Figure 3.8 Total anomalous pulmonary venous connection

Early management involves ventilation, correction of acidosis, and prostaglandin infusion. Definitive treatment is primary repair of the anomalous venous connection on cardiopulmonary bypass. The long-term prognosis is good if the baby survives surgery.

Persistent fetal circulation

Also known as persistent pulmonary hypertension of the newborn, this type of non-structural heart disease seems to be getting less common. It may complicate respiratory distress syndrome, meconium aspiration, or diaphragmatic hernia, or may be precipitated by polycythaemia, hypoglycaemia, etc. It occasionally affects well-grown term babies with no obvious underlying cause. There is usually no tachypnoea and no sign of heart failure. The pulmonary second sound is loud and there may be a soft systolic murmur. On chest X-ray the heart size is normal and the lung fields are clear. The ECG is normal. The diagnosis is made by exclusion of other forms of cyanotic heart disease by echocardiography but is obviously strongly suspected in the presence of a possible precipitating cause. Management is conservative: correct any identified precipitating abnormality (such as polycythaemia or hypoglycaemia); give oxygen and, if necessary, use artificial ventilation to produce a low Paco$_2$ and thus reduce pulmonary resistance. Severe cases may require prolonged ventilation and sometimes tolazoline infusion (see below).

Prostaglandin E$_2$ in the management of cardiac lesions in neonates

Prostaglandin E$_1$ and E$_2$ are used to dilate the arterial duct. Duct-dependent cardiac abnormalities fall into two main groups:

1. Cyanotic lesions (mainly critical pulmonary stenosis, pulmonary atresia and tricuspid atresia) where pulmonary blood flow depends upon continuing patency of the duct.
2. Acyanotic lesions (mainly coarctation syndrome and interrupted aortic arch) where perfusion of the lower half of the body is maintained by the duct.

Prostaglandin may also be used where adequate systemic and pulmonary mixing is dependent upon ductal flow, such as in transposition of the great arteries prior to balloon septostomy.

Cyanotic neonates

In cyanotic infants prostaglandin is effective in improving oxygenation when clinical deterioration has been precipitated by duct closure. It will increase pulmonary blood flow via the duct and will also dilate the pulmonary vascular bed. In transposition of the great arteries, both before and after balloon atrial septostomy, prostaglandin may be used to increase aorta to pulmonary artery shunting through the duct. This is balanced by an increase in left to right atrial shunting and mixing of oxygenated and de-oxygenated blood is improved. In cyanotic infants prostaglandin is most effective when the initial Pao_2 is low; when the birth weight is below 4 kg; and during the first four days of life.

Acyanotic neonates

Many infants with coarctation of the aorta or interrupted aortic arch will respond to prostaglandin infusion with improved perfusion of the lower limbs, return of femoral pulses, increased urine output, and less tendency to metabolic acidosis. Age, initial Pao_2 and birth weight are less critical factors than in cyanotic heart disease. The full effect of prostaglandin in acyanotic lesions may take 3–4 h to appear, whereas in cyanosed babies the response is usually seen within 30 min.

Intravenous treatment

Both prostaglandin E_1 and E_2 will produce dilatation of the duct. The infusion is given intravenously. No increased benefit is obtained by administration into a pulmonary or systemic artery.

Most centres now use prostaglandin E_2. Mix 500 μg of prostaglandin E_2 in 500 ml 5% dextrose. The infusion rate is 0.6 ml/kg dose of 0.01 μg/kg/min. Recommended doses of prostaglandin E_1 in the literature are 0.05–0.1 μg/kg/min but experience has shown that lower doses are usually equally effective.

Several side-effects have been associated with prostaglandin infusion but few are serious enough to warrant stopping the drug. The most important is respiratory depression and apnoea; this is most likely to happen in infants less than 2 kg and in those with cyanosis, and is almost certainly dose related. It is uncommon with the dose that we use but resuscitation facilities must be close at hand. Low-grade pyrexia, drowsiness and poor feeding are frequent, but minor, problems. Cutaneous vasodilatation was seen in the days of intra-aortic infusion but it is not a problem with intravenous infusion. Increased risk of sepsis is a theoretical risk but most sick babies receive penicillin and gentamicin and all postoperative babies are given flucloxacillin, so this is unlikely to be a practical problem. Convulsions, jitteriness and diarrhoea are occasional side-effects of intravenous treatment.

Starting therapy

Prostaglandin therapy is usually started shortly after admission, often before an exact anatomical diagnosis has been reached, and is discontinued once the patient has undergone a surgical procedure or once the duct has been shown to be closed. It is not widespread policy to recommend starting prostaglandin infusion before transfer of babies to the regional paediatric cardiological centre but occasionally this is necessary. As long as the accompanying paediatrician is aware of the possiblity of sudden apnoea, there should be no particular problem in transferring babies on a prostaglandin infusion.

Oral treatment

Prostaglandin infusion is generally a temporary measure – to improve the infant's condition before he undergoes coarctectomy, balloon septostomy, aortopulmonary shunting, etc. Occasionally, and especially with pulmonary atresia, oral prostaglandin may be given over a longer period so that the baby is more mature and heavier by the time he comes to surgery. The oral dose of prostaglandin E_2 is 50 µg/kg/h given hourly via a nasogastric tube. Obviously the baby has to remain in hospital while this treatment is in progress and it is best for him to remain in the regional paediatric cardiac unit as duct closure may occur on this treatment. If it does not respond to an intravenous infusion of prostaglandin, urgent surgery will be necessary. Oral prostaglandin is given by making an oral suspension of dinoprostone (Prostin E_2) tablets to form a suspension containing 100 µg/ml. It must be shaken vigorously before being measured out and a fresh suspension is made up every 6 h.

Tolazoline in paediatric cardiology

Tolazoline is a histamine-like compound related to phentolamine. It has three main groups of effects:

1. *Histamine-like*. This includes both pulmonary and peripheral vasodilatation (by direct action on smooth muscle) and stimulation of gastric secretion.
2. *Sympathomimetic*. The most prominent effect is cardiac stimulation, producing tachycardia and arrhythmias.
3. *Parasympathomimetic*. This includes stimulation of the intestinal tract, an action blocked by atropine.

Tolazoline is used mainly to produce acute pulmonary vasodilatation. The commonest indications are:

1. Persistent fetal circulation or pulmonary hypertension in the neonate, both as a primary disease and complicating respiratory distress syndrome, etc.
2. During cardiac catheterisation for investigation of left-to-right shunts with severe pulmonary hypertension to determine whether the pulmonary vascular disease is potentially reversible.
3. In the postoperative management of patients with pulmonary hypertension who are prone to pulmonary hypertensive crises.

The single intravenous dose is 1–2 mg/kg. Be prepared for systemic hypotension which may require colloid infusion. For maintenance treatment an intravenous infusion of 1–2 mg/kg/h may be used. Mix 50 mg tolazoline/kg body weight in 50 ml dextrose 5% and give at 1–2 ml/h.

Tolazoline is mainly excreted unchanged by the kidneys so beware of its use in renal failure.

Unwanted effects are largely an inevitable part of the drug's action, and are dose related and therefore not necessarily avoidable. They include:

- systemic hypotension
- nausea
- vomiting
- abdominal pain
- increased gastric acid production
- hyperperistalsis
- diarrhoea
- stimulation of salivation and lacrimation
- sweating
- chill
- apprehension.

Although some of the gastrointestinal effects may be reduced by cimetidine or ranitidine, both drugs probably also reverse the pulmonary vasodilator action and should not be used.

Conditions presenting with heart failure in infancy

Cardiac failure in infancy generally presents with breathlessness (especially during feeds), poor feeding, failure to thrive, and sweating. The symptoms are similar, whatever the underlying cause. Acute exacerbations of heart failure in children with known heart disease must be distinguished from respiratory infections, bronchiolitis, etc. Physical examination will reveal tachypnoea, intercostal recession and sweating. There may be evidence of failure to thrive. Hepatomegaly is a much more reliable sign in this age group than elevation of the venous pressure. Other features on examination depend mainly on the cause of the cardiac failure.

The treatment of heart failure will also depend largely on the underlying cause but certain general principles apply.

1. *Diuretics* are the mainstay of medical treatment. They are usually given orally but may be given intravenously to sick children (the intravenous dose of frusemide is 0.5–1 mg/kg). For maintenance treatment in this unit we routinely use a combination of chlorothiazide and spironolactone (20–40 mg/kg/day and 2–4 mg/kg/day respectively). Other units will use frusemide (1–3 mg/kg/day) with potassium supplements (KCl 1–2 mmol/kg/day).
2. *Digoxin.* The debate about the effectiveness of digoxin in heart failure continues. It is certainly reasonable to use it when myocardial contractility is impaired and many paediatricians still use it when heart failure results from a left-to-right shunt. The dose/kg is variously quoted on a sliding scale but is best administered as $200 \, \mu g/m^2/day$. Care is needed with dosage in renal impairment, hypokalaemia, etc.
3. *Tube feeding* is often helpful if there is failure to thrive or a feeding problem. It guarantees a fluid and calorie intake and saves energy.
4. *Nursing* in a sitting position is advice often quoted but largely out of date. It predates more effective treatment for heart failure. Whilst it may be helpful in some cases, it is largely unnecessary and some babies are unhappy and uncomfortable in this position.
5. *Vasodilators.* These are often used intravenously if there is an acute problem but may be appropriate orally for chronic heart failure where there is no immediate prospect of surgery. Captopril or enalapril are the two most often used and both are angiotensin converting enzyme inhibitors. The dose of captopril is 0.25 mg/kg/day, increasing as necessary to a maximum of

6 mg/kg/day and given as two or three doses daily. Captopril is not recommended with renal impairment or hyponatraemia. Beware of hypotension at the start of treatment.
6. *Further treatment* depends largely on the clinical situation and on the underlying abnormality. More aggressive treatment for heart failure includes administration of oxygen, consideration of artificial ventilation, infusion of inotropic drugs, etc.

Ventricular septal defect

Most defects causing symptoms are large or are associated with other cardiac abnormalities. While small to moderate defects classically have a pansystolic murmur with a thrill, large defects may have little or no murmur if there is pulmonary hypertension or may be accompanied by a loud mid-diastolic murmur if the shunt is large. The chest X-ray generally shows cardiomegaly with pulmonary plethora and the ECG may show left ventricular hypertrophy or biventricular hypertrophy. The diagnosis will be confirmed on echocardiography which will demonstrate the position and size of the defect. Full assessment will include a search for other ventricular septal defects, coexisting ASD, PDA, coarctation, etc. Management includes general advice for heart failure given above. If symptoms continue, the choice is between pulmonary arterial banding and closure of the septal defect. The choice will be governed largely by the size and age of the child and also by the type of defect but most centres these days would prefer early closure of the VSD, where possible.

Patent arterial duct

This is a common cause of heart failure in infants, even those born at term. Classical signs include collapsing or bounding pulses, clinical left ventricular hypertrophy, a continuous murmur, often with a systolic 'rattle'. The chest X-ray will show cardiomegaly and pulmonary plethora. The ECG often shows left ventricular hypertrophy. The diagnosis is confirmed by Doppler echocardiography and cardiac catheterisation is unnecessary. The management is ligation or division of the duct.

Truncus arteriosus

The aorta and the pulmonary artery originate in a common trunk. This usually presents between four and ten weeks of age with heart failure. On examination the pulses are bounding or collapsing and there may be clinical biventricular hypertrophy. The second heart sound is single and the systolic and diastolic murmurs should be distinguished from VSD plus PDA, VSD with aortic regurgitation, etc. The chest X-ray will show mild cardiomegaly, an absent main pulmonary arterial shadow, and pulmonary plethora. The ECG will show biventricular hypertrophy.

The prognosis for this lesion is still not good, although surgical results are improving. If the truncal valve is stenosed or regurgitant then the outlook is generally poor. The plan is to perform repair in severe cases within the first six months of life, these children being very prone to early postoperative pulmonary hypertensive crises. Because of the small conduit in a small child, later replacement of the conduit is necessary.

Aortopulmonary window

The presentation is similar to truncus arteriosus or ventricular septal defect with a large ductus. Signs are those of pulmonary hypertension with a large left to right shunt at great artery level.

Echocardiographic demonstration of a connection is sometimes difficult but is easier now that Doppler is available. Angiography will confirm the situation if there is any doubt.

Total anomalous pulmonary venous connection

The obstructed forms (usually with infradiaphragmatic connection) generally present in the neonatal period. More common are the non-obstructed types, often with supracardiac connection. The physical signs resemble a large atrial septal defect with right ventricular hypertrophy or enlargement, a widely split fixed second sound, a pulmonary ejection murmur, and a tricuspid diastolic flow murmur. The chest X-ray will show cardiomegaly and, if the connection is supracardiac, a large upper mediastinal shadow or 'snowman heart'. The ECG usually shows right axis deviation with right ventricular hypertrophy or right bundle branch block. The diagnosis these days is confirmed on echocardiography. Treatment involves surgical anastomosis of the pulmonary veins to the left atrium.

Cardiomyopathy

This may occur at any age but, if presenting in infancy, the outlook is often poor. Specific physical signs are few although there is often a murmur of mitral regurgitation and a third heart sound. The chest X-ray shows marked cardiomegaly, sometimes with pulmonary oedema. The ECG sometimes shows left ventricular hypertrophy and often shows ST segment or T wave abnormalities. The diagnosis is established by echocardiography which shows a dilated, poorly contracting left ventricle with no structural heart disease. It is important to identify any correctable underlying abnormality, such as anomalous left coronary artery (see below) or incessant atrial tachycardia. The treatment of cardiomyopathy is generally as outlined above, with vasodilators, diuretics, digoxin, etc.

Univentricular atrioventricular connection

A variety of rare and complex abnormalities may cause heart failure in infancy. They are mostly forms of tricuspid atresia or double inlet ventricle with unrestricted pulmonary flow causing heart failure. Initial treatment is palliative and depends on the exact anatomical arrangement.

Fontan is the definitive procedure.

Anomalous origin of the left coronary artery

The left coronary artery takes its origin from the main pulmonary artery. This anomaly usually presents with heart failure around 2–3 months when the normal fall in pulmonary artery pressure has precipitated myocardial ischaemia and infarction. There is often a murmur of mitral regurgitation. The chest X-ray shows cardiomegaly. The ECG usually shows a transmural anterolateral myocardial infarction. The diagnosis may be confirmed by echocardiography but cannot be excluded by this technique and angiography is still sometimes necessary. Treatment is urgent translocation of the left coronary to the aorta.

Atrioventricular septal defect

Two forms may present with heart failure in infancy. The first is a *complete* atrioventricular septal defect (previously known as atrioventricular canal). Roughly half of these children have Down's syndrome. There may be signs of pulmonary hypertension, high pulmonary flow and atrioventricular valve regurgitation. The electrocardiogram is helpful in that it almost always shows a leftward QRS axis. The diagnosis is confirmed by echocardiography. As surgical results of repair of this lesion have improved, there has been less enthusiasm for palliation by pulmonary artery banding. Postoperative pulmonary hypertensive crises are common.

The second type presenting in infancy is a *partial* atrioventricular defect (ostium primum ASD) with significant mitral valvular regurgitation. The signs and investigations are similar to above except that there is no ventricular septal defect. If conservative treatment of heart failure is ineffective, surgery is indicated but repair of the left atrioventricular valve may present difficulties.

Surgical treatment is usually through the right atrium. The common mitral and tricuspid leaflets are separated, the mitral valve is repaired, the ASD and VSD closed with a common patch and the valve leaflets attached to it.

Conditions presenting with a murmur

Many children with congenital cardiac lesions are symptomatic and are dealt with above, but others may still have significant abnormalities requiring surgical correction.

Ventricular septal defect (see also p. 167)

Most VSDs are small and many of these will close spontaneously. However, some children with large defects remain asymptomatic. The chest X-ray will give some indication of the size of the shunt. If there is cardiomegaly and pulmonary plethora the defect is likely not to be small. If the electrocardiogram shows right ventricular hypertrophy one should suspect pulmonary hypertension, right ventricular outflow obstruction, or double outlet right ventricle. If there is clinical evidence of a moderate to large left-to-right shunt, cardiac catheterisation may be indicated. The dividing line between surgical and conservative management is unclear but many children with $Qp:Qs$ greater than 2 or 2.5:1 will be recommended to undergo surgical closure. Non-invasive and invasive investigations should assess pulmonary arterial pressure and look for evidence of subaortic stenosis, mitral regurgitation, subpulmonary stenosis, etc.

Patients with ventricular septal defects not undergoing surgery should of course be advised about antibiotic prophylaxis against infective endocarditis.

Atrial septal defect

Most children with this lesion are asymptomatic. The clinical diagnosis is usually easy. There is evidence of right ventricular hypertrophy or enlargement with a fixed split second sound, a moderate pulmonary ejection murmur, and often a tricuspid diastolic murmur. The chest X-ray may show cardiomegaly, with pulmonary artery enlargement and a small aorta, as well as pulmonary plethora. The ECG will show right axis deviation and right bundle branch block. Left axis deviation indicates an ostium primum defect. The diagnosis will be confirmed on echocardiography. The pulmonary venous connection should be assessed, as hemi-anomalous pulmonary venous connection is not an uncommon association.

The anatomy may be:

1. Secundum type: in the mid-portion of the septum.
2. Primum type: associated with mitral and tricuspid valve defects.
3. Sinus venosus: high in the septum and associated with partial anomalous pulmonary venous drainage.
4. Coronary sinus.

The most common type is the secundum type and surgery is indicated if there is significant shunt (Qp:Qs ratio > 1.5:1.0). Some centres operate on ASD routinely because of the possibility of further complications: arrhythmias, paradoxical embolism, late pulmonary damage and right heart failure.

The primum type is more serious because of its association with anomalies of the atrioventricular valves, as part of the spectrum of atrioventricular septal defect.

In the sinus venosus type the right superior pulmonary vein is connected with the superior vena cava.

Every case should be assessed individually to decide if direct suture or patch with repair of associated anomalies if necessary. Surgical complications are heart block, arrhythmias, endocarditis and failure of repair.

Pulmonary stenosis

Critical pulmonary stenosis presents with cyanosis in infancy. Most other children are asymptomatic. The severity of the valvular stenosis can be assessed clinically: those with mild stenosis have no clinical right ventricular hypertrophy, a constant ejection click and, at most, a moderate ejection murmur; more significant stenosis will only have an expiratory ejection click, which will be rather earlier, diminution of the pulmonary second sound, a loud murmur with a thrill, and right ventricular hypertrophy on the ECG. The most severe cases have no ejection click at any stage of breathing. In almost all centres surgical valvotomy has been replaced by percutaneous balloon valvotomy. This is indicated when the valve gradient is greater than 30 or 40 mmHg. The occasional patient with a dysplastic pulmonary valve (as in Noonan's syndrome, etc.) may require enlargment of the right ventricular outflow with insertion of a patch.

Aortic valvular stenosis

This is a common lesion. Most patients are asymptomatic and assessment is aimed at identifying those requiring treatment before symptoms occur. Clinical assessment of the severity of stenosis is aided by the ECG (which may indicate left ventricular hypertrophy or show ST segment or T wave abnormalities) and Doppler echocardiography (which will assess the transvalvular gradient). Patients with evidence of significant stenosis should undergo cardiac catheterisation to measure the valvular gradient. Surgical valvotomy has traditionally been advised in those with a catheter gradient greater than 70 mmHg, even in the absence of symptoms. It has recently been largely supplanted by percutaneous balloon dilatation. The indications for dilatation are similar to those for surgery. Dilatation is advised in all patients with symptoms and in those with a pressure gradient greater than 50 or 60 mmHg. Patients with severe aortic regurgitation or those in whom balloon dilatation is unsatisfactory may require consideration for aortic valvular replacement.

In subvalvular stenosis, resection of the fibromuscular membrane will relieve the obstruction.

Other alternatives in specific cases are: aortic valvular replacement; Konno procedure (aortoplasty enlarging the aortic annulus and the ventricular septum with patch closure and aortic valvular replacement); left ventricle to aorta conduit.

Supravalvular aortic stenosis

The indications for treatment are similar to aortic valvular stenosis. Echocardiography and aortic angiography will distinguish this lesion from valvular stenosis. Assessment should include right heart catheterisation as coexisting pulmonary arterial stenosis is frequent. Pulmonary arterial stenosis tends to improve spontaneously while supraventricular aortic stenosis is progressive. The treatment of choice is surgical patch enlargement of the ascending aorta.

Hypertrophic cardiomyopathy

This is a rare familial condition characterised by gross left ventricular hypertrophy. The two main complications are left ventricular outflow obstruction and arrhythmias. The prognosis in patients with symptomatic or haemodynamically significant arrhythmias seems to be improved by treatment with amiodarone. Symptoms of chest pain or syncope in patients with significant outflow obstruction may respond to treatment with propranolol. Surgical myectomy is occasionally required. Care is taken during the operation not to cause aortic or mitral valvular regurgitation or to induce complete heart block.

Congenital cardiac disease in the adult

This is a rapidly developing aspect of 'paediatric' cardiology, partly because of increasing awareness and therefore increasing recognition of some asymptomatic lesions, but mainly because improved surgical results over the past 10 or 20 years have produced a generation of survivors of previously unsurvivable cardiac abnormalities. This has great implications for the provision and management of resources and other factors such as genetic counselling. When those adolescents become young adults they need to know the long-term implications of their residual heart disease, to be given advice about contraception, pregnancy and the likelihood of their children being affected. They also need advice about employment, life insurance, prophylactic antibiotics, etc.

Several types of congenital cardiac disease are seen in young adults.

New referrals

A surprising number of patients with congenital heart disease come to light for the first time in teenage or young adult life. A secundum atrial defect is generally picked up because of the presence of a murmur, or may present with heart failure or atrial arrhythmias in the third and fourth decade. Coarctation of the aorta is usually diagnosed when hypertension is detected, either during insurance or employment medicals in men, or during assessment for contraception or pregnancy in women. Other new diagnoses made not infrequently include persistent arterial duct, milder forms of Ebstein's anomaly, congenitally corrected transposition of the great arteries without a haemodynamically significant lesion, and arrhythmias such as Wolff–Parkinson–White syndrome.

Long-term follow-up of benign lesions

Patients with small ventricular septal defects, mild pulmonary stenosis (PS), mild aortic stenosis, and other lesions not requiring surgery form most of this group. Non-progressive lesions such as mild PS or a small VSD probably do not require long-term specialist follow-up. Patients with aortic valvular disease are probably best kept under occasional review, as are those with minor but more significant lesions which will be unfamiliar to a general practitioner or a general physician, or for that matter to an adult cardiologist.

Inoperable lesions

Included amongst this group are patients with Eisenmenger's syndrome, pulmonary atresia and VSD with poorly-developed pulmonary arteries, and other more complex lesions, some of which may have been palliated during childhood. This is a growing group of patients who will need sympathetic handling and will need to be given advice about heart or heart–lung transplantation, as well as general aspects of management covered above.

Survivors of corrective surgery

Over the next few years we shall see many more patients in this group. 'Correction' of abnormalities such as Fallot's tetralogy, transposition of the great arteries, and so on, is now becoming routine and most patients will survive into early adult life. They will be kept under long-term follow-up, partly so that long-term results can be assessed and also because they risk the development of late problems which may go unrecognised in a general medical or adult cardiological clinic. Complex operations such as a Fontan procedure, a Senning operation or a Rastelli operation may each be associated with its own particular problems. Any patient with a conduit or prosthetic valve is at risk from late obstruction. Many of these procedures are also associated with late arrhythmias or late sudden death. Almost all patients with congenital heart disease will need to be given antibiotic prophylaxis against infective endocarditis.

Paediatric postoperative care (general)

Post-cardiac surgery intensive care of infants and children is integrated with pre-operative assessment, intra-operative procedures and long-term follow-up. Greater emphasis is placed on intensive monitoring and manipulation of cardiovascular physiology.

Transfer from operating theatre to ITU

Patients are most vulnerable during this journey. The anaesthetist will usually employ hand ventilation. ECG monitoring and transcutaneous oximetry are employed throughout the transfer. Drug infusions, particularly those of inotropes and other vasoactive drugs, must be maintained using battery-powered infusion pumps. Drains must be connected appropriately and it is vital to ensure that infants and small children do not get cold during the transfer.

Routine postoperative monitoring

Monitoring of heart rate, heart rhythm, systemic arterial pressure, central venous pressure, central and peripheral temperatures and saturation via an oximeter are established. Left atrial and pulmonary arterial pressures will be monitored in selected patients. Urine output and the amount of fluid in the drain will be measured at least hourly. Blood gases, haematocrit, blood clotting and serum potassium will be checked frequently. Once the patient is settled, a chest X-ray should be performed.

The surgeon must detail the type of operation, the duration of bypass, any residual cardiac abnormalities and the site of drains, pacing wires, etc.

Ventilation

Simple cases will have been extubated in theatre and will be breathing spontaneously on return to the ITU. They require monitoring of respiration rate, heart rate, colour and, if possible, oxygen saturation. Most will be on morphine infusion and will be observed for evidence of respiratory depression. Many other children and almost all neonates require a period of artificial ventilation postoperatively.

Uncuffed nasotracheal tubes are used routinely, fixed firmly to avoid accidental displacement. The type of ventilator and its

Table 3.1 Endotracheal tube sizes

Age	Size (mm)
Newborn	3
1 y	3.5
3 y	4
6 y	5
8 y	6
10 y	7
14 y	8

settings are decided by the child's age, size and blood gases. The rate, pressure, and Fio_2 are adjusted as required to keep the acid–base balance and $Paco_2$ normal. A low Pao_2 may be acceptable in children with cyanotic heart disease. Oxygenation may be aided by PEEP (positive end-expiratory pressure) but high levels are avoided as they impede venous return and impair cardiac output.

While all children are sedated, usually with morphine, during ventilation, few are paralysed unless there is a particular problem (e.g. pulmonary hypertensive crisis) which makes this necessary. If the haemodynamic and pulmonary situation is satisfactory, the ventilation is gradually reduced, monitoring the blood gases and oxygen saturation. Most patients will spend at least a short period on CPAP (continuous positive airway pressure) before being extubated. Following extubation, infants should be placed in a headbox connected to humidified oxygen. Children will usually tolerate a facemask; if not, the oxygen can be administered by a feeding-tube with two holes placed under the nostrils.

Postoperative physiotherapy is routine. In ventilated infants physiotherapy is usually combined with hand-bagging and endotracheal suction.

If the child deteriorates after extubation, ventilation will need to be reinstituted. The cause is often retained secretions or may be pulmonary congestion, phrenic nerve palsy, etc.

With a correctly fitting endotracheal tube it is usually possible to continue ventilation for several weeks without particular problems. Subglottic oedema may be produced in some children with prolonged ventilation and may be eased by administration of intravenous dexamethazone before extubation. Tracheostomy is rarely required these days.

Postoperative fluid balance

Normal fluid requirements for the neonate are:

- day 1   60 ml/kg/24 h
- day 2   75 ml/kg/24 h
- day 3   90 ml/kg/24 h
- day 4   120 ml/kg/24 h
- day 5+ 150 ml/kg/24 h.

These rough guides will need to be adjusted depending on the clinical situation. The fluid input should be increased by up to 30 ml/kg/day for babies nursed under a radiant heater, receiving phototherapy, or with pyrexia. The input will also need to be adjusted in patients with renal failure, cardiac failure, or electrolyte imbalance.

Normal fluid requirements in infants and children are:

- < 10 kg   100–120 ml/kg/day
- 10–20 kg   90–120 ml/kg/day
- > 20 kg   50–90 ml/kg/day.

Sodium and water are often retained after surgery. This does not usually present problems after closed surgery but after open cardiac surgery fluid restriction may avoid circulatory overload. Monitoring of all input should include drugs, line flushes, etc. Fluid balance will also be judged by weighing if possible, particularly in patients in intensive care for more than a few days. Insensible loss can only be guessed but becomes more important in patients with fever, diarrhoea, necrotising enterocolitis, or those being nursed under a radiant heater.

Postoperative colloid and crystalloid infusions are usually judged independently. The amount of colloid or blood depends on circulatory balance and will be judged from the systemic arterial pressure, central venous pressure, left atrial pressure, peripheral temperature and losses via drains. The total crystalloid input is computed separately and is adjusted in the light of urine output, biochemical results, etc. The total, including drugs and line flushes, is restricted to:

- day 0   500–750 ml/m²/day
- day 1   750–1000 ml/m²/day
- day 2 1000–1250 ml/m²/day.

Hourly equivalent levels are:

- day 0 20–30 ml/m²/h
- day 1 30–40 ml/m²/h
- day 2 40–50 ml/m²/h.

Dextrose 5% is used as a standard. Potassium supplements will be necessary (as detailed below). Sodium is usually not necessary in the newborn or immediately postoperatively but otherwise is added as below.

The normal requirements for sodium and potassium are as follows:

- neonate   2.5–3.5 mEq/kg/day ⎫ depending on the clinical
- infant < 10 kg 2.5–3.5 mEq/kg/day ⎬ situation and plasma
- child 10–20 kg 2.0–2.5 mEq/kg/day ⎬ levels.
- child > 20 kg   1.5–2.0 mEq/kg/day ⎭

Aim to keep the serum potassium between 4.0 and 4.5 mmol/litre. Increased potassium loss is common following cardiac surgery, especially in patients receiving diuretics, and is compounded by pre-operative depletion. Renal loss of potassium is reduced in patients with renal failure, infection, and acidaemia.

The normal serum sodium is 135–145 mmol/litre. Hyponatraemia is generally an indication of water overload rather than sodium depletion. Hypernatraemia may result either from dehydration or from over-zealous sodium administration, often as the bicarbonate, to correct acidaemia in sick neonates.

Renal function is monitored by 24-hourly urinary output, electrolytes, urea and creatinine, and osmolality. The normal urine output should be greater than 0.5 mg/kg/h or greater than 300 ml/m^2/24 h. For further details of normal and abnormal renal function see p. 184.

Inotropic support

Cardiac preload, afterload and myocardial contractility can all be manipulated independently. Many of the drugs will influence more than one of these factors. Normal cardiac output (measured clinically and indirectly), rate, rhythm, filling pressures, afterload (pulmonary and systemic arterial pressures) and myocardial performance are the aim. Filling pressures are maintained by colloid infusion; if high, they are an indication of impaired myocardial function or, in some instances, are an inevitable result of the type of surgery (e.g. Fontan). Inotropes and vasodilators are used to affect afterload and myocardial contractility. Contractility is often impaired postoperatively as a consequence of bypass, cardioplegia, or direct surgery on the ventricular myocardium.

Dobutamine

This is a synthetic beta stimulant. It improves cardiac output by increasing contractility and reducing afterload. Unlike dopamine it does not increase afterload at higher doses. There is generally some increase in heart rate with no direct effect on blood pressure, although this may increase a little as the cardiac output rises.

Dopamine

This is a naturally-occurring alpha and beta stimulant. At low doses ($2-5\,\mu g/kg/min$) there is a direct dopaminergic effect on renal blood flow and glomerular filtration. At intermediate doses ($5-10\,\mu g/kg/min$) the beta effect is dominant and is similar to the action of dobutamine. At higher doses (greater than $10\,\mu g/kg/min$) the peripheral alpha effect produces systemic vasoconstriction, increasing afterload and myocardial oxygen consumption, so doses in this range are therefore generally avoided. At higher doses dopamine will produce arrhythmias.

Adrenaline

This has both alpha and beta effects and is used to increase heart rate, blood pressure and myocardial contractility. Higher doses will produce hypertension and arrhythmias and the drug increases myocardial oxygen consumption.

Isoprenaline

This is a synthetic beta-stimulant. It increases heart rate rather than contractility and is a vasodilator in both the pulmonary and systemic circulations. It is used mainly to counteract bradycardia.

Glyceryl trinitrate (nitroglycerine)

This is a vasodilator which, at moderate doses, mainly affects venous tone and preload but at high doses also reduces systemic and pulmonary arterial resistance. Higher doses may produce hypotension and tachycardia.

Sodium nitroprusside

A vasodilator with a dominant effect on arterial pressure. It is used to reduce afterload when left ventricular function is impaired and

Table 3.2 Paediatric doses of emergency intravenous drugs

Drug	Concentration	Dose/kg	Neonate (3.5 kg)	2 months (5 kg)	6 months (7.5 kg)	12 months (10 kg)	8 years (25 kg)	14 years (50 kg)
Adrenaline 1:10000	100 µg/ml	10 µg/kg	0.35 ml	0.5 ml	0.75 ml	1.0 ml	2.5 ml	5.0 ml
Atropine	600 µg/ml	15 µg/kg	0.1 ml	0.15 ml	0.2 ml	0.25 ml	0.5 ml	1.0 ml
Bicarbonate 8.4%	1 mmol/ml	0.5 mmol/kg	1.0 ml	2.5 ml	3.5 ml	5.0 ml	15.0 ml	25.0 ml
Calcium gluconate 10%	100 mg/ml	10 mg/kg	0.35 ml	0.5 ml	0.75 ml	1.0 ml	2.5 ml	5.0 ml
Diazepam	5 mg/ml	200 µg/kg	0.4 ml	1.0 ml	2.0 ml			
Defibrillation	1 J/kg			5 J		10 J	25 J	50 J

Table 3.3

Drug	Supplied as	Add	To	Infusion rate (ml/h)	Dose (µg/kg/min)
Adrenaline	1 mg in 10 ml (1:10000) 1 mg in 1 ml (1:1000)	300 µg/kg	50 ml 5% D	1.0–3.0	0.1–0.3
Dobutamine	250 mg in 10 ml	30 mg/kg	50 ml 5% D	0.2–1.0	2.0–10.0
Dopamine	200 mg in 5 ml	30 mg/kg	50 ml 5% D	0.2–1.0	2.0–10.0
Isoprenaline	2 mg in 2 ml	300 µg/kg	50 ml 5% D	0.5–3.0	0.05–0.3
Morphine	10 mg in 1 ml	1 mg/kg	50 ml saline	1	20 (µg/kg/h)
Nitroglycerine (GTN)	5 mg in 2 ml	3 mg/kg	50 ml 5% D	0.1–0.5	0.1–0.5
Nitroprusside	50 mg in 2 ml	3 µg/kg	50 ml 5% D	0.5–3.0	0.5–3.0
Prostacyclin	500 µg in 50 ml diluent	30 µg/kg	50 ml saline	0.5–2.0	5.0–20.0
Prostaglandin E_2	750 µg in 0.75 ml	500 µg	500 ml 5% D	0.6 (ml/kg/h)	0.01
Tolazoline	25 mg in 1 ml	25 mg/kg	25 ml 5% D	1–2	1.0–2.0 (µg/kg/h)

is also particularly useful for control of paradoxical hypertension following resection of coarctations. It has a very short half-life. The dose should be increased and decreased slowly rather than abruptly. Overdose will produce hypotension and compensatory tachycardia.

Analgesia and sedation

Analgesia is important, not only on humane grounds but also because the postoperative progress will be smoother, and hypertension, tachycardia, etc. are minimised if the child is comforted. Adequate analgesia should be given during procedures such as removal of chest drains, and problems such as pulmonary hypertension, renal failure requiring dialysis, etc.

Morphine infusion

Morphine 1 mg/kg body weight is mixed with 50 ml normal saline. An infusion given at 1 ml/h provides a dose of 20 μg/kg/h. This should be preceded by a loading dose of 200 μg/kg/h. The dose can then be modified by increasing the infusion rate or by giving intravenous top-up doses of 100 μg/kg as necessary. Respiratory depression presents no problem in ventilated children but respiration and transcutaneous oxygen saturation should be monitored in spontaneously-breathing children. Marked respiratory depression or apnoea can be reversed by naloxone 5–10 μg/kg given as a single intravenous dose. This can be repeated once if not effective. Naloxone has a shorter half-life than morphine, so further doses may be necessary. Morphine is excreted only slowly by neonates and therefore has a prolonged effect. An apnoeic and unresponsive neonate who has had morphine many hours before may respond dramatically to naloxone.

Short-term analgesia for removal of drains, etc. can often be provided satisfactorily by administration of nitrous oxide by inhalation.

Many children appear to have surprisingly little pain postoperatively but oral analgesia should be prescribed routinely once intravenous analgesia is discontinued. Paracetamol elixir is the safest and easiest routine drug; it contains 120 mg in 5 ml. The dose is:

- 0–1 years   60–120 mg
- 0–5 years 120–240 mg
- 6+ years 240–480 mg.

Paracetamol tablets will be suitable for older children and suppositories are also available. It is worth considering a regular prescription because if analgesia is only given 'as required' there may be a delay in administration because the nurses are busy. Analgesia not given until there is sufficient pain will be less effective. For the first nights after operation it may be appropriate to top up this type of analgesia with a dose of morphine or Omnopon.

Postoperative antibiotics

In Freeman we use flucloxacillin in all patients for 2–5 days (oral flucloxacillin is very unpalatable and often children refuse to take it!). No attempt is made to use broad spectrum antibiotics which increase the number of multiresistant organisms found on routine cultures. Other antibiotics are given as bacterially indicated for suspected or proven infections.

Nutrition

The normal energy requirements of children are as follows:

- neonate   110 kcal/kg/day
- infant < 10 kg   100 kcal/kg/day
- child 10–20 kg   75–100 kcal/kg/day
- child > 20 kg   45–75 kcal/kg/day

Calorie requirements are increased dramatically by cardiac surgery and also by fever and pre-operative malnutrition. Our aim is to recommence feeding as soon as possible postoperatively. Wherever possible feeding is enteral, usually by nasogastric tube. Most proprietary brands of baby milk provide about 110 calories in 150 ml so no supplements are necessary.

Parenteral nutrition

The aim is to provide an adequate intake of fluid, electrolytes, carbohydrate, amino acids, fat, calories, trace elements and vitamins. Dextrose 5% contains only 20 calories per 100 ml and even 10% dextrose is barely an adequate source of calories. Intravenous feeding should be performed through a sterile central line with a filter in the circuit. The line is not used for any other purpose.

The pharmacy in many hospitals undertaking neonatal or infants' intensive care will provide a standard pre-prepared TPN infusion which can be modified when appropriate, to include more potassium, etc. Further details of intravenous feeding are given in Roberton (1986) and Insley (1986).

Specific general postoperative neonatal problems

Temperature control

Neonates, especially if premature or underweight, cannot maintain their temperature adequately and need to be nursed in a 'thermoneutral' environment. An incubator provides the best control of temperature and humidity but is incompatible with the access necessary for good postoperative care. Babies, therefore, are usually nursed under radiant heaters and compensation is made for their increased insensible water loss. Hypothermia is most likely to develop during transfer to and from theatre, and during operation or cardiac catheterisation. Significant hypothermia will increase the mortality in sick neonates.

Hypoglycaemia

Sick neonates with congenital cardiac disease often develop hypoglycaemia. This is easily detected and controlled by regular testing with BM sticks and infusion of 10% dextrose if the reading is < 3 mmol/litre. If it is out of proportion to the cardiac problem or unusually difficult to control, consult Roberton (1986).

Jaundice

This is common but usually not a serious problem. Special note should be taken if:

1. Jaundice develops rapidly on the first day of life. This may be due to rhesus or ABO incompatibility (check Hb, blood group, Coomb's test); a red cell abnormality such as spherocytosis (check family history and blood film), or congenital infection (do TORCH screen and platelet count).
2. Jaundice develops rapidly after 24 hours. Check for infection. Check blood group and Coomb's test.
3. Jaundice perists for longer than 10 days. Exclude infection, hypothyroidism and galactosaemia. Most often this is a normal finding in a breast-fed infant.

Treatment of unconjugated jaundice with phototherapy is indicated if the bilirubin rises above 340 µmol/litre in a term baby.

Postoperative pyrexia and infection

Pyrexia is common after all forms of cardiac surgery, particularly those involving cardiopulmonary bypass. It is most often non-infective but investigations should include cultures of blood, urine, and tracheal secretions, measurement of the white blood count, and urine microscopy. It is treated by tepid sponging and by administration of paracetamol and, if appropriate, with a vasodilator. It is worth cross-checking that the pre-operative nose, throat and urine culture, etc. were all negative.

Pyrexia late in the recovery period may be due to:

1. *Early onset of endocarditis.* Fortunately this is less common in children than adults undergoing valve surgery. If peri-operative flucloxacillin is given, infection with staphylococcus should be avoidable. The diagnosis is established by repeated blood cultures and may be supported by the finding of vegetations on echocardiography although this is not common at this stage. Unusual organisms such as candida or pseudomonas may be grown on culture. An appropriate course of antibiotics is necessary and re-operation is occasionally indicated.
2. *Post-pericardiotomy syndrome.* This is a diagnosis of exclusion of infective causes and is an inflammatory reaction to the operation, generally presenting 2–6 weeks postoperatively. It causes fever and chest pain. Physical examination may disclose raised venous pressure, pleural or pericardial rub. The chest X-ray may show a pleural effusion or cardiomegaly, and echocardiography may identify a pericardial effusion. The ESR or CRP and the white blood count are usually raised. Treatment includes aspirin and is conservative. Steroid treatment is rarely indicated.
3. *Persisting undiagnosed fever.* Keep looking for an infection. The extent of the investigation depends upon the clinical situation.

Renal failure

Preservation of adequate renal function depends on the maintenance of normal cardiac output, systemic blood pressure, intravascular volume and tissue oxygenation. Some children with abnormal kidneys respond badly to the normal, strict fluid restriction after bypass.

Urine output is monitored, usually with an indwelling catheter early after surgery, though expression of the bladder in neonates is relatively simple. If the urine output is low, check that the catheter is not blocked. Oliguria is defined as a urine flow less than 0.5 ml/kg/h or less than 300 ml/m^2/24 h.

Oliguria usually complicates low cardiac output. In addition to the usual measures, dopamine is said to have a specific 'dopaminergic' effect on the kidneys in a 'renal' dose of 2–5 µg/kg/min.

It is important to establish whether a patient with oliguria has prerenal failure or established renal failure. Measure the plasma and urinary elecrolytes, urea, creatinine and osmolality. Table 3.4 shows how results will help to distinguish between prerenal and renal failure.

Table 3.4

	Pre-renal failure	Renal failure
Urine Na$^+$ (mmol/l)	>20	<10
Urine: plasma creatinine	>20	<10
Urine osmolality (mosmol/kg)	>500	<350
FE Na (%)*	<1%	>2%

*Fractional excretion of sodium is calculated as: [Na] urine/[Na] plasma × [creatinine] plasma/[creatinine] urine. It is no use in patients who have received diuretics, i.e. most of those in intensive care.

Prerenal failure is reversible. Correct hypotension and low cardiac output if possible. Give i.v. frusemide 1 mg/kg. If there is no response, give a larger dose of 3–4 mg/kg. Set up a dopamine infusion at 2–5 µg/kg/min. Consider an infusion of mannitol.

If these measures fail, or if the results indicate that the patient has established acute renal failure, further management will be in conjunction with a paediatric nephrologist. It is important to monitor the serum potassium. Dangerous hyperkalaemia can be temporarily corrected by giving i.v. calcium gluconate 10% (0.3 ml/kg) and/or administration of 1 unit insulin and 4 g dextrose/kg body weight. Correct acidaemia with sodium bicarbonate. Hyperkalaemia is one of the indications for peritoneal dialysis.

Ideally, any decision regarding the institution of peritoneal dialysis will be made in conjunction with the paediatric nephrologist; it is employed early if there is marked fluid overload or hyperkalaemia. Details of the fluid cycle, volume, installation and dwell times, etc. will vary from patient to patient. It is vital to maintain an adequate calorie intake.

In the 'diuretic' recovery phase which follows oliguria in acute renal failure, be prepared to maintain water, sodium and potassium input to avoid dehydration and hypernatraemia or hypokalaemia.

Fits and acute brain injury

Postoperative fits are always a worrying development because they sometimes indicate cerebral damage with a poor outlook. Overall the prognosis after an isolated postoperative fit is good.

Fits in the newborn

Take blood to check the glucose, sodium, calcium and magnesium. Give i.v. phenobarbitone 10–20 mg/kg. If this is ineffective, give diazepam 1–2 mg. If fits continue, paraldehyde 1 ml i.m. or i.v. or phenytoin 10-20 mg/kg i.v. may be indicated. Once fits are under control give a maintenance dose of phenobarbitone 5 mg/kg/day. Remember that fits may, rarely, be caused by meningitis, so consider the need for a lumbar puncture. If there is a possibility of cerebral damage related to catheterisation or surgery arrange a cerebral ultrasound scan.

Febrile convulsions

These should be largely preventable if postoperative pyrexia is kept in check. Give phenobarbitone or diazepam as above.

Fits related to cerebral ischaemia

These may complicate cardiac surgery, or rarely, catheterisation, and may be caused by inadequate cerebral perfusion or by cerebral emboli. The fitting is controlled with phenobarbitone and/or diazepam. If there is evidence of generalised brain injury, consider the following additional measures:

1. Hyperventilation to reduce the $Pa\text{co}_2$ to around 3–3.5 kPa. Increase the $F\text{io}_2$ as appropriate.
2. Intravenous mannitol and/or frusemide as for treatment of acute renal failure.
3. Some authorities would recommend dexamethazone.
4. Generalised cooling will reduce cerebral metabolism.

Specific cardiothoracic postoperative paediatric problems

Postoperative arrhythmias

Minor variations of cardiac rhythm are common after both open and closed operations. So long as they do not impair the cardiac output and do not produce marked bradycardia or tachycardia they are best ignored. Atrial and ventricular ectopic beats are perhaps encountered most often, are usually benign and do not require treatment. If they are frequent, check the serum potassium and calcium and correct as appropriate. Also check the position of the central venous line on the chest X-rays as this may produce ectopics if inserted too far.

Complete atrioventricular block

With improvements in surgical technique and better understanding of the position of atrioventricular conduction tissue in various cardiac abnormalities, this has become a less frequent complication. It most often occurs in smaller children undergoing closure of ventricular septal defect, repair of complete atrioventricular septal defect, or repair of tetralogy of Fallot and sometimes complicates complex surgery. In any patient at risk the surgeon will usually insert temporary atrial and ventricular pacing wires. Pacing is instituted as necessary to maintain an adequate heart rate. Atrial wires enable sequential atrioventricular pacing to be done. Ventricular demand pacing is satisfactory unless the cardiac output is poor, in which case insertion of a transvenous temporary electrode to the right atrium should be considered. The AV delay is usually set at around 150 ms. Postoperative complete atrioventricular block is often temporary and no decision about permanent pacing is necessary for two or even three weeks. If the heart block resolves, follow-up should include 24-hour ECG tape monitoring to identify any children at risk. If it persists, permanent pacing will be necessary in most or all children.

Junctional tachycardia

This is the commonest form of significant SVT in the early postoperative period. It usually occurs after open heart surgery in infancy, such as VSD closure, Senning operation, repair of total anomalous pulmonary venous connection, etc. It both results from and contributes to the presence of a low cardiac output and acidaemia, etc. The diagnosis is suspected when there is a regular, narrow QRS tachycardia 200–350/min (the QRS may be wide if the operation has produced bundle branch block) and is confirmed by the finding of ventriculoatrial block, i.e. slower dissociated P waves. These may sometimes be easier to identify by direct recording of the ECG from atrial pacing wires. Some patients with this arrhythmia do not have AV block. Junctional tachycardia is an automatic arrhythmia and generally resolves within 48 hours or so, but may cause significant haemodynamic impairment. It is refractory to underdrive pacing, overdrive pacing, DC cardioversion and many drugs. Management includes correction of underlying hypotension, acidosis, etc. and avoidance of tachycardia-inducing inotropic drugs where possible. Digoxin is ineffective. Verapamil may be dangerous. Drugs which may be effective include flecainide and propafenone. Both these are negatively inotropic and must be given with great caution and with colloid infusion to counteract hypotension. Intravenous amiodarone (5 mg/kg) may sometimes be effective. Systemic cooling may also help to control the tachycardia.

Atrial arrhythmias

Postoperative atrial flutter is uncommon but is usually easy to identify. If there is 1:1 or 2:1 conduction, diagnosis may be difficult and is then facilitated by intravenous administration of adenosine (see below) or by recording an electrogram from temporary pacing electrodes. Atrial flutter will usually respond to overdrive atrial pacing or electrical cardioversion. Digoxin, disopyramide, or amiodarone may help to maintain sinus rhythm if the arrhythmia is recurrent. Disopyramide for atrial flutter should only be given to a digitalised patient.

Atrial fibrillation may complicate the Fontan operation. It then usually indicates an unsatisfactory haemodynamic situation and results from right atrial hypertension and distension. It often causes further haemodynamic deterioration. It may respond, at least temporarily, to DC shock but attention must be paid to the underlying haemodynamic problem.

Other supraventricular tachycardias

Other significant supraventricular arrhythmias are uncommon postoperatively, especially when they have not occurred pre-operatively. Patients with Wolff–Parkinson–White syndrome or other accessory pathways, undergoing open cardiac surgery, will usually have their pathways identified and divided at surgery.

Types of SVT not considered under specific headings above will usually respond to underdrive or overdrive atrial pacing, if available. Adenosine is the drug of choice, producing marked slowing of AV conduction but having a very short half-life. The initial dose is 50 µg/kg, increasing if ineffective by 50 µg/kg/dose to a maximum of 250 µg/kg. Most episodes of SVT will also respond to DC shock, if this is necessary.

Ventricular tachycardia

The potassium level should be checked. If there is doubt about the diagnosis, intravenous adenosine (see above) may help to distinguish VT (which will be unaffected) from SVT (which will be terminated) or atrial arrhythmias (which will demonstrate AV block). Atrial dissociation on the surface ECG or the atrial electrogram will also aid the diagnosis of VT. VT will usually respond to DC shock or intravenous lignocaine (dose 1 mg/kg); it may also respond to ventricular pacing undertaken by an expert.

Hypotension and low cardiac output

Systemic arterial pressure is easy to measure, while cardiac ouput is not. The two variables are related but blood pressure is not a good indicator of cardiac output.

The normal or acceptable blood pressure varies with age so that a systolic pressure of 50 mmHg may be quite satisfactory in the newborn but would give cause for concern in an older child. The level of blood pressure is not important if tissue perfusion is adequate, especially that to the brain, heart and kidneys.

Table 3.5 Guide to causes of low cardiac output and action to be taken

Underlying cause	Clues	Action
Hypovolaemia	Low atrial pressure Cool periphery	Transfuse
Poor cardiac function	High atrial pressure Cool periphery	Inotropic support
Septicaemia	Low arterial pressure Warm periphery	Blood culture Antibiotics Inotropic support
Tamponade	High atrial pressure Cool periphery	Echocardiogram Urgent surgery

Cardiac output is best assessed clinically from the peripheral temperature (or the difference between the central and peripheral temperature) and from the urine output. A low cardiac output from any cause will be indicated by a low mixed venous oxygen saturation and often by acidaemia. Cardiac output can be measured by the Fick principle, by thermodilution techniques, and by Doppler echocardiography.

Bleeding

Postoperative bleeding is an uncommon but potentially serious problem. It will be made worse by pre-operative polycythaemia, thrombocytopenia, clotting disturbances, and administration of salicylates or anticoagulants. In severely polycythaemic children, consideration should be given to pre-operative venesection. Bleeding will also be worse after long, difficult operations and re-operations.

The normal blood volume is:

- 85 ml/kg in infants < 10 kg
- 80 ml/kg in children 10–20 kg
- 75 ml/kg in children > 20 kg

Blood losses via the drains are monitored regularly and are replaced, with blood if the haematocrit is below 35%, and with plasma above 40%. In the face of bleeding, check the ACT (or other index of anticoagulation) and, if prolonged, give protamine 250 µg/kg. Consider surgical re-exploration if:

1. The blood loss exceeds 10% of the blood volume in any hour.
2. Blood loss exceeds 5% of the blood volume per hour more than three hours after return from theatre.

Pneumothorax

This is a not uncommon finding on a routine chest X-ray, especially after the removal of chest drains, but it is rarely large enough to cause a problem. However, pneumothorax in the neonate may produce a sudden and dramatic unexplained deterioration. If the diagnosis is suspected, examine the chest with a cold light and, if in doubt, insert a chest drain.

Chylothorax

This results from damage to the thoracic duct, usually during an operation performed via an upper left thoracotomy. It most often complicates coarctectomy or duct ligation in infancy. It causes continuing drainage via the chest drain or a pleural effusion after the drain is removed. The fluid is clear if the child is fasting and is cloudy if he is being fed. Diagnosis is confirmed by the finding of lymphocytes or fat cells in the fluid on microscopy.

The management is to make sure that an adequate fluid intake is maintained, that electrolyte balance is normal, and that a high calorie intake is given. It is best to use a high medium-chain-triglyceride milk (such as Progestimil). If the fluid loss continues, the child may rapidly become wasted and is in danger of serious electrolyte imbalance so, if the situation is not improving, the chest should be re-explored. Surgeons are often hesistant to re-open the chest but re-operation is usually effective, even though a leak may not be identified.

Phrenic nerve palsy

All prospective surveys reveal a high incidence of phrenic palsy which often goes unrecognised. One must have a high index of suspicion and be alerted by the finding of a high hemidiaphragm on chest X-ray or by difficulty in weaning from ventilation. Phrenic palsy may complicate operations performed by thoracotomy or sternotomy. The diagnosis is confirmed by the finding of paradoxical movement of the diaphragm during spontaneous respiration. This is best assessed by fluoroscopy but may also be confirmed by echocardiography. It is not possible to confirm the diagnosis while the child is being ventilated.

Management is usually conservative especially in those with adequate cardiopulmonary reserve. If progress is slow, or if weaning from ventilation proves impossible, plication of the diaphragm should be considered.

Postoperative systemic hypertension

Systemic arterial hypertension is an uncommon but undesirable complication of cardiac surgery. It increases left ventricular afterload and, therefore, myocardial oxygen consumption, and may also impair cerebral function in infants who have lost cerebral autoregulation following cardiopulmonary bypass.

Systemic hypertension most commonly results from pain which should be suspected especially when there is an associated tachycardia. The blood pressure will usually respond to administration of adequate analgesia.

Postoperative hypertension is also commonly seen after resection of coarctation. Recent papers have shown that this can be prevented by pretreatment with oral propranolol, given in a dose of 2–3 mg/kg/day. Paradoxical hypertension following coarctectomy is best managed acutely with an infusion of sodium nitroprusside. The infusion is begun at 0.5 µg/kg/min and is increased up to 3 or 5 µg/kg/min, or occasionally more, depending on the effect. The nitroprusside is continued until oral beta-blocker treatment can be reinstituted where necessary.

Labetalol is an alternative to nitroprusside but experience of its use in children is limited.

If the hypertension observed is unexpected and cannot be easily explained, it is important to check the calibration of whatever type of measurement is being employed and to cross-check the pressure with another method. Put not thy faith in electricity.

Pulmonary hypertension

This has recently been recognised as a significant cause of early postoperative mortality in infants at risk. A pulmonary hypertensive crisis begins with a paroxysmal increase in pulmonary vascular resistance. This increases the pulmonary arterial pressure, often to a level higher than systemic pressure. The right ventricle is then unable to maintain pulmonary flow and the cardiac output and sytemic pressures fall. Before this series of events was recognised, and before appropriate monitoring was used, there was no sign of trouble until the systemic pressure fell, by which time the situation was often irreversible.

Infants most at risk are those between 3 and 12 months undergoing repair of lesions which have large left-to-right shunts and pulmonary hypertension, such as VSD, transposition with VSD, complete atrioventricular septal defect, truncus arteriosus or aortopulmonary window.

As with most aspects of postoperative care, prevention is better than cure. All children at risk are monitored and early intervention will often prevent a deterioration. If possible, lines will be inserted at the time of surgery to monitor left atrial and pulmonary arterial or right ventricular pressure.

Prevention of a crisis

Much postoperative care will be routine, with special attention being paid to maintenance of normal blood gases and avoidance of hyperpyrexia. Monitoring of pulmonary arterial pressure will provide early warning of a crisis. Susceptible patients are paralysed, sedated and ventilated. Aim to keep the Pao_2 above 13 kPa, the $Paco_2$ less than 4 kPa and the mean PA pressure at less than half the mean systemic arterial pressure. Further hepful preventative measures include avoidance of dopamine and adrenaline, with use of dobutamine and/or isoprenaline instead, if necessary. Patients will usually have received phenoxybenzamine in theatre, which is often continued postoperatively. The dose is 0.5–1 mg/kg every 8 hours. Unless there are particular respiratory problems, routine chest physiotherapy is best avoided in the early stages.

Treatment of a crisis

If the pulmonary arterial pressure rises above a predetermined level (50 or 75% of systemic arterial pressure) further steps are necessary as follows:

1. Increase the Fio_2 to 1.0 and hand ventilate.
2. Give prostacyclin 5–10 ng/kg/min through the PA line.
3. Ensure effective sedation and paralysis.
4. Other pulmonary vasodilators, such as tolazoline, may be helpful.

Failures of management

Success does not always reward the righteous. For instance, filling pressures are often higher following repair of Fallot's tetralogy because of poor right ventricular compliance, etc. Optimal haemodynamics after the Fontan operation also differ from any other type of operation. If things are not going well in the early postoperative period, despite model management, it is important to remember the possibility of an operative failure. The surgeon may conclude that revision of the operation or further surgery is necessary.

Following aortopulmonary shunts, especially those using a synthetic graft, persisting hypoxaemia may suggest occlusion or thrombosis of the shunt. Shunt murmurs are often difficult to hear in the first day or so. If the shunt appears not to be functioning, it may improve with colloid infusion or haemodilution. Doppler echocardiography or angiography will show whether the shunt is patent.

Persisting failure after VSD closure may be due to ventricular impairment or may be due to dehiscence of the patch which can be assessed with Doppler echocardiography.

Poor cardiac output following repair of Fallot's tetralogy may have several causes. Among them is persisting right ventricular outflow obstruction. If the situation cannot be improved rapidly, this may be an indication for re-operation.

Following the Mustard or Senning operation, early caval obstruction or pulmonary venous obstruction is now rare but not unknown.

Unsatisfactory haemodynamics after the Fontan operation usually results from poor patient selection. Low cardiac output, high right atrial pressure, and atrial fibrillation are poor prognostic signs but, despite this, management is usually medical. In some cases there may be reason to consider taking down the Fontan operation and performing palliative aortopulmonary shunt.

Nursing care of children after cardiac surgery

All children undergoing open heart surgery, and many children having closed surgery and cardiac catheterisation, will be cared for in the paediatric intensive care unit.

Preparation

The preparation of the patient's bed before his admission is the first step. The size and weight of the child are important when deciding what the baby will be nursed on, e.g. neonates will be nursed on an overhead-radiant babytherm-Drager; children weighing over 5 kg on an adult-sized cardiac bed.

The following equipment is required on the bed which will be sent to theatre to transfer the child to ITU:

- portable ECG monitor with leads;
- at least two battery operated syringe pumps to continue inotropic support during transfer;
- space-blanket to maintain body temperature;
- drainage clamps (the drains should not be clamped during transfer);
- oxygen cylinder with appropriately-sized hand-ventilation set to ventilate the child until settled on the machine in the unit;
- pacing box and leads.

At the bedside there will be triscope monitoring equipment for ECG, arterial pressure and right atrial pressure. Apparatus for endotracheal suction is situated behind the bed, with low-pressure suction which will be attached to indwelling drains. Two oxygen flowmeters are checked to ensure they are connected properly and in working order. The number of syringe-pumps required will depend on the child's condition and at least four of them should be available after open heart operation. One volumetric pump should be required for delivering the maintenance intravenous therapy.

Ventilation

The patient is usually ventilated mechanically. The choice of ventilator will depend upon the size of the child. Smaller children are nursed on either Sechrist or Bird ventilators, which are both pressure-cycled. Older children will have Servo ventilators, with a preset minute volume. The anaesthetist sets the minute volume, pressures, inspiratory and expiratory times. He will have to make sure that the alarms are switched on. Soon after the child is settled on the ventilator, an arterial blood gas analysis enables finer adjustment of the ventilator.

The patient's colour and chest movement are observed. Ventilator pressures and heart rate are recorded. Transcutaneous Po_2/Pco_2 monitoring is often more useful than the arterial line. Most children are sedated when on the ventilator with a morphine infusion set according to body weight, with extra, as necessary, as morphine boluses combined with midazolam or diazepam. Endotracheal suction is performed two-hourly and as necessary. The amount and type of secretions will be recorded.

Early detection of chest infection is vital. A daily sputum is sent to the laboratory for Gram stain, culture and sensitivity.

The ventilator temperature is kept at 37.5–38°C, well-humidified to enable the secretions to be aspirated easily. If the secretions are too tenacious, 0.5 ml 0.9% sodium chloride solution into the endotracheal tube during physiotherapy may break them up.

The child will have a chest X-ray as soon as he returns from theatre and each morning routinely. As the humidification system is a closed circuit on the paediatric ventilators, it is not necessary to change the ventilator circuit every day.

The physiotherapist should visit him four times daily. If there are areas of consolidation, hand ventilation during physiotherapy may be required, and when the patient is cardiovascularly stable he will be nursed from side-to-side.

The endotracheal tube is held in place by a headpiece which consists of latex foam roll and elastoplast. Nursing care of both tube and headpiece is extremely important. The connector end attached to the endotracheal tube must be secured far enough from the nose to make sure it does not cause pressure sores or necrosis in a child who may need longer term ventilation. As the headband may cover bony parts on the skull, the patient will need frequent positional change.

As the child's condition improves, the amount of mechanical ventilation required will reduce. The children on Sechrist or Bird ventilators will gradually have their respiratory rate and pressures reduced until they are able to breathe spontaneously on CPAP. Then the gases are frequently checked, the general perfusion and oxygenation observed, and once the medical staff are satisfied that the patient is coping he can be extubated.

Following extubation, oxygen is delivered by various methods depending on size, age and how cooperative the child is. Older children may tolerate a face mask connected either directly to flowmeters or given via an inspiron to humidify the gas. If the child cannot tolerate a mask, nasal spectacles, or a suction catheter with holes cut in it, placed under the nostrils and taped to the child's face, may be more acceptable.

Babies are nursed in a headbox, which is a perspex box placed over the child's head, and humidified oxygen is administered. An oxygen analyser is placed in the headbox to monitor the percentage of oxygen being delivered. An 'apnoea mattress' will be placed under the child to warn the nurse should the patient fail to breathe.

Blood gas analysis continues at regular intervals until the condition improves. Once it is stable, the transcutaneous monitor is discontinued as well.

Cardiovascular monitoring

Recognition of abnormal rhythms is essential, since they can be life threatening (VF), can reduce the cardiac output (tachycardia, bradycardia), or indicate electrolyte imbalance (ventricular ectopics).

Nursing staff must be familiar with normal pressures and traces in order to provide accurate information and detect deviations from the normal promptly. The child's clinical condition should bear some resemblance to the figures on the screen. A basic knowledge of the equipment is indispensable. The correct position of the transducer in order to have an accurate zero is basic. Patency of the cannula is maintained by using a continuous sodium chloride flushing system and particular care is taken not to kink or displace the cannula. The circulation distal to the cannula site is checked regularly since embolisation may occur.

When inotropes are discontinued from the right atrial line, a flush must be taken from it in order to remove any residual drug. It is also important not to give bolus drugs through lines infusing inotropes, for the same reason.

The left atrial line needs particular care because injection of air may occur. Removal of these lines should be carried out at least one hour prior to removing mediastinal drains.

All cannula sites should be kept clean and free from infection. Dressings need to be changed at least once daily, and should be applied in such a way that the cannula is not kinked or pulled. Lines may need to be changed if the site shows inflammation or if the patient has a persistent pyrexia of unknown origin. Line-tips are sent to the laboratory for bacteriology, culture and sensitivity.

Central temperature might be a problem in small children. Infants are nursed with overhead heaters and have a space-blanket until the central temperature reaches 36°C.

Postoperative pyrexia of 38°C is common a few hours after surgery. If the pyrexia is persistent, blood culture, urine specimen and tracheal secretions are sent to the laboratory for investigation.

Peripheral temperature is an indicator of cardiac output. It is monitored by the nurse at regular intervals and can be reported as warm, cool, cold. Probably the important point is the peripheral movement of skin warming, which should be assessed by the same person.

Drains

Mediastinal drains are inserted during the operation, connected to underwater seal and applied to suction (10 mmHg). The amount of drainage is recorded every half-hour. Blood loss is replaced according to the packed cell volume (PCV), as blood products may be required rather than whole blood.

'Milking' drains may be required to ensure patency. A sudden cessation of drainage may indicate cardiac tamponade if other signs of sudden low cardiac output are present.

Fluids

Fluid input and output are strictly recorded. The child's maintenance infusion, flushes and drugs are recorded hourly. Urine output is carefully documented as well as any additional losses, particularly from the gastrointestinal tract.

The most common electrolyte imbalance is hypokalaemia.

Regular monitoring of serum potassium levels and replacement therapy are essential. Additional care must be taken when children have a large diuresis in response to diuretic therapy. Four-hourly reflochecks are monitored in children to ensure they are receiving an adequate glucose intake. Daily levels of calcium and magnesium are also checked in these children, who are prone to convulsions.

Feeding

Following surgery, it is important to introduce feeding at an early stage, aiming to resume what the child was having pre-operatively, i.e. breast milk, SMA, Cow and Gate, etc.

If the patient is extubated he will be given small amounts of feed frequently and gradually returned to his normal feeding pattern. If there is difficulty, a reasonable compromise should be to give him as much as he can manage from the bottle without becoming breathless and tired, the remainder being given via a nasogastric tube.

Babies remaining ventilated for longer than 24 hours will require nasogastric feeding. Mothers who breast-feed will be asked to express breast milk and this may be given through the nasogastric tube.

Feeding may commence as a continuous feed or with boluses, usually given every two hours depending on which the child tolerates best. Once feeding starts, the fluid balance must be reviewed as the maintenance intravenous therapy will need to be decreased when nasogastric feeding has been established. The tube is aspirated 2–4-hourly and the patient should be nursed side-to-side or on his tummy, with his head slightly elevated; never on his back, a position which risks the aspiration of stomach contents.

Equipment used for feeding must be thoroughly cleaned, usually in hot soapy water and refilled with a Milton solution. Equipment should be washed thoroughly and then submerged in the Milton solution for at least one hour before being used again.

If enteral feeding is not possible or contraindicated then intravenous feeding is used. The pharmacy will make up a paediatric solution to the calculated specification. The feeding-line is usually inserted into the subclavian vein and will be used for feeding only. The usual biochemical tests will be taken daily: urea and electrolytes, 24-hourly; liver function tests, 3 times weekly; and blood glucose according to each particular situation.

Hygiene

The baby is nursed on alternating sides. His position and nappies are changed 2–3-hourly and all nursing procedures will respect the patient's rest. The nappies are carefully weighed in order to keep an accurate fluid balance. Mouth and eye care take place when the child's position is changed. Oropharyngeal suction is performed and the mouth is cleaned with weak effervescent mouthwash solution. The eyes are cleaned by instilling normal saline or hypromellose. It may be necessary to tape the eyes to keep them closed in order to avoid corneal abrasion in curarised or unconscious patients.

Transcutaneous Po_2 probes may also be changed when other care is being performed. These probes require changing every 2–3 hours to avoid burning the skin. Surgical incisions will be redressed once daily. If there is any sign of inflammation or infection, samples for culture and sensitivity will be sent. The wound's condition will be recorded in the notes.

Relatives

Parents of children requiring intensive care are extremely anxious. Prior to surgery they should be given the opportunity to visit the Unit so they can meet some of the staff and adapt to the environment. The nurse can explain some of the equipment at the bedside in simple terms. Visiting is unrestricted. Accommodation for the parents and access to catering facilities near to the ITU are ideal. When the patient returns from theatre the parents are informed about his condition. All procedures are properly explained beforehand. Relatives are encouraged to take part in the child's care.

Respiratory medicine

Respiratory physiology

The lungs are the organs where respiratory gases are exchanged. They are complex, compressed within the thoracic cavity and conceal a massive surface area of which the smallest basic unit is an alveolous. The internal lining membrane is the interface between the gaseous external environment and the 'fluid milieu interior': across it are exchanged the volatile products of respiration and of metabolism. A complicated, dynamic partnership of checks and balances between pulmonary and cardiac function is governed by biochemical feedback loops, centrally-mediated reflex arcs and brain stem activity, to optimise this exchange under the constantly-changing conditions of human existence. Assessment is of 'snapshots' of data, which in turn are summations or extrapolations from the many processes of respiration. Pathophysiological assessment depends on interpreting such results in the light of conceptual models and clinical findings.

The respiratory membrane

The fundamental model is the air–blood interface, the respiratory membrane. It represents an air-filled sac (alveolus) separated from a blood vessel (pulmonary capillary circulation) by a single-layer, permeable interstitium. The alveolar surface is humidified, moist and in contact with atmospheric air. The vessel contains blood from the pulmonary artery which is to be replenished with oxygen and scrubbed of some of its carbon dioxide during the time it is in close contact with the alveolus and before it enters the pulmonary vein. The basic laws of gas physics apply, so the motive force for exchange is the partial pressure (or tension) differential each gas (oxygen, carbon dioxide and nitrogen) exerts across the respiratory membrane. The higher partial pressure of oxygen in atmospheric air drives oxygen into the blood. The alveolus is the first stage of a progressive fall (oxygen cascade) in oxygen partial pressures that favours the transport of oxygen from air to cellular mitochondria: its pressure differential across the respiratory membrane is maintained by the carriage of oxygen molecules away from the lungs for use during aerobic metabolism. A reverse gradient exists for carbon dioxide. Because carbon dioxide is a waste product of metabolism which is only present in very small amounts in the atmosphere, the pressure gradient is from the blood to the alveolus, from where its molecules are exhaled during normal, tidal respiration. Nitrogen, being metabolically inert, is in equilibrium between the alveolus and the tissues and its movement is only of import because of a physical role in maintaining alveolar distension, or under abnormal conditions, notably during the breathing of oxygen-rich mixtures or in deep-sea diving.

Oxygen cascade

The oxygen cascade starts with a step down in partial pressure in the alveolus from that in atmosphere because of the presence of water vapour, exerting its own partial pressure. A second fall, often greatly exaggerated in disease, is recognised as occurring because of an imbalance between ventilation and perfusion. To define this, the simple respiratory membrane model has to be modified to include end-points on a representative spectrum. One end represents an alveolus that is collapsed but has a capillary supply derived from the pulmonary artery; that is, it is perfused but not ventilated. The other end represents a reverse situation, that is, a ventilated alveolus with no blood supply. The ratio derived from these two factors (V/Q ratio) is therefore mathematically zero in the former, and infinite in the latter. A low V/Q ratio is manifest as hypoxaemia because it is indicative of blood remaining desaturated as a result of traversing oxygen-poor alveoli; it is described as shunted blood. More correctly, it is physiological shunting as opposed to anatomical or true shunting, which is the addition of non-pulmonary to systemic arterial blood, as for example, that from bronchial veins, Thebesius' veins or, classically, the right-to-left shunting of cyanotic heart disease. All these vascular shunts, summated, may contribute to measurable arterial hypoxaemia. This addition of desaturated blood, with a similar oxygen content to that of mixed venous blood, has given rise to the concept of venous admixture of systemic arterial blood. These shunts are usually quantified by expressing their amount relative to cardiac output (Qs/Qt).

A very high V/Q ratio represents wasted ventilation that may contribute little or nothing to respiration. It is referred to as physiological dead space when 'anatomical' dead space – that is, the conducting airways from mouth to respiratory bronchioles – is included. Because of the extreme solubility of carbon dioxide, its removal is almost independent of blood flow but a total absence of flow to ventilated alveoli, or an increase in dead space, is manifest as carbon dioxide retention or hypercapnia. A similar analogy to shunting is often drawn and the wasted ventilation is usually expressed as the ratio of dead space to tidal ventilation (Vd/Vt).

The influence of pressure

The various intrathoracic pressures, alveolar and vascular, are close to atmospheric pressure. The interactive relationships influence the distribution of blood flow. Small changes in any of the levels may have profound effects on respiratory function. Conceptual models must take account of them as changes are manifest as falls in the oxygen cascade.

Pulmonary areas (West zones) can be delineated from the differentials between the pulmonary capillary pressures and alveolar pressure that may exist at any one time. In some areas of the lung, notably those influenced by gravity (upright posture, lung apices), the pressure in the alveolus may tend to exceed pulmonary arterial capillary pressures, so that no blood will flow. Although such alveoli will have high V/Q ratios, they functionally represent maldistribution of blood flow and, in effect, contribute to ventilation–perfusion mismatch and venous admixture. In dependent parts of the lung, again because of gravitational effects, the intrapleural pressure may be less 'negative' than at the apices, with the result that some alveoli may remain collapsed during quiet ventilation. These perfused but not ventilated alveoli also contribute shunted blood, although a natural mechanism, labelled as hypoxic pulmonary vasoconstriction, acts to minimise its effect by diverting perfusion away from hypoventilated areas.

Measurement of respiratory physiological data

In clinical practice the visible end result of many of the events that take place in the lungs are changes in arterial blood gas tensions. Ventilation–perfusion mismatch and shunting manifest as a change in the partial pressure of oxygen between alveolus and arterial blood (A–a gradient). In theory, a similar widening of this gradient may represent a physical bar to the passage of oxygen across the interstitium between alveolus and capillary (e.g. by pulmonary oedema or pulmonary fibrosis). In practice, most of any demonstrable arterial hypoxaemia represents ventilation–perfusion mismatch and local shunting. For carbon dioxide tension the key is alveolar ventilation; any fall in effective ventilation will show up as hypercarbia, excessive alveolar ventilation will result in hypocarbia.

It is evident that measurements of alveolar events are necessary to unravel these complex pulmonary relationships. In practice, they are studied by the data obtained from inspired and expired gases and from mixed venous and arterial blood sampling. Several mathematical formulae, based on assumptions and fundamental derivations, can be used to numerate pulmonary physiology in normal and diseased states. The important formulae are:

Bohr equation

$$Vd/Vt = \frac{(P_{aCO_2} - P_{ECO_2})}{(P_{aCO_2})}$$

Shunt equation

$$Qs/Qt = \frac{C_{IO_2} - C_{aO_2}}{C_{IO_2} - C_{vO_2}}$$

Alveolar gas equation

$$P_{aO_2} = P_{IO_2} - \frac{P_{aCO_2}}{R}$$

The transport of oxygen

The biological transporter for oxygen is haemoglobin. Very little oxygen is carried in any other form, so that haemoglobin is a virtual monopoly reservoir. The local chemical environment influences the oxygen–haemoglobin relationship favouring binding at high oxygen tensions and its release at low oxygen tensions. The relationship between the partial pressure (or tensions) of oxygen and the amount of oxygen that can be carried by the blood is delineated by the oxygen saturation (or dissociation) curve for haemoglobin (Figure 4.1). From the plot of the curve it can be seen that a flat portion occurs when haemoglobin is carrying its maximum amount of oxygen and that it will do this over a wide physiological range of oxygen tensions but that at a level of about 80% saturation the pattern changes, so that a small change in oxygen tension may result in a rapid decline in the amount of

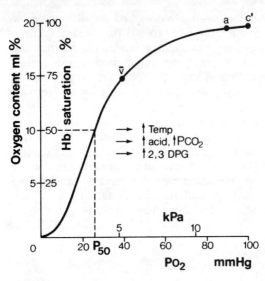

Figure 4.1 The oxygen dissociation curve

oxygen carried. At levels below 60% saturation, symptomatic evidence of hypoxia occurs.

Blood pH, temperature, concentration of 2,3-diphosphoglyceric acid (2,3-DPG) and carbon dioxide partial pressure influence the relationship and may 'shift' the curve either to the right or the left. Any shift can be defined by the P_{50} (the partial pressure of oxygen at which the haemoglobin is 50% saturated). Alkalosis, hypothermia, a low 2,3-DPG concentration, e.g. stored blood, and hypocarbia increase the tendency for haemoglobin to retain its oxygen at the expense of tissue oxygenation; the P_{50} is less, the saturation curve shifted to the left. Right shifts, e.g. acidosis, hypercarbia, pyrexia, represent a climate favourable for the release of oxygen from its carrier.

The oxygen content per millilitre of arterial blood can be derived from saturation, the haemoglobin concentration, and the knowledge that each gram of haemoglobin, when fully saturated, carries 1.3 ml oxygen:

arterial O_2 content = saturation × haemoglobin concentration × 1.3

Importantly, the total quantity of oxygen available for exchange per minute (sometimes known as the oxygen flux) can be calculated by multiplying the arterial content by the cardiac output. The calculation of the oxygen flux can be useful in pathological states because the role and relationship of each of these measurable variables (the oxygen saturation, the haemoglobin concentration and the cardiac output) in the delivery of oxygen can be defined.

The transport of carbon dioxide

Carbon dioxide is very soluble in blood and active chemically under physiological conditions. A carbon dioxide dissociation curve shows that content can change from 0 to 50 ml/100 ml blood over a narrow spectrum of partial pressure because it is so readily converted into alternative chemical forms in the blood:

1. In solution in the plasma (3–5%).
2. In combination with ammonium radicals of haemoglobin-carboxyhaemoglobin and other blood proteins (2–10%).
3. As bicarbonate (80%) in a reaction catalysed by carbonic anhydrase present in red cells.

These reactions tend to be reversed by the chemical environment, that in the tissues favouring the formation of these alternative forms, and that in the pulmonary circulation favourable for its release for diffusion into alveoli.

Regulation of respiration

Several regions in the mid-brain are recognised as constituting parts of a respiratory centre. One of these has an intrinsic, automatic ability to institute rhythmical ventilation but is open to modulating influences from a variety of sources, including information from other parts of the centre. The major influence in health is the carbon dioxide tension in the blood, with chemoreceptors in the respiratory centre functioning as though set to maintain $Paco_2$ level in a physiological range, with any increase precipitating hyperventilation. Oxygen lack is a late stimulant which is mediated by chemoreceptors in the aortic and carotid bodies. Other important intermediaries that act through the respiratory centre and induce reflex respiratory changes include intrathoracic stretch-receptors (Hering–Breuer reflex), proprioceptors (e.g. in exercise) and pain. All initiate increased drive of the respiratory muscles and a greater depth, force and rate of rhythmical activity.

The mechanics of respiration

Intrathoracic pressure is subatmospheric so that quiet inspiration is almost passive, the driving atmospheric pressure opening the airways and expanding the chest wall to accommodate the tidal volume of air. The resistance to expansion of the alveoli, the elasticity of pulmonary tissues and the weight of the chest wall are the main resistive forces to be overcome. In health, the alveoli do not need to be forcibly re-expanded during inspiration; their complete collapse during expiration is prevented by a surface tension that is maintained by a secreted surface lipoprotein known as surfactant. Intercostal and diaphragmatic muscular contractions aid in overcoming the resistive properties of pulmonary tissue and chest wall. Equalisation of oral and alveolar pressures, and responses of pulmonary stretch-receptors initiate expiration, which is again largely passive and brought about by an elastic recoil of the lungs, which is conducted at a controlled rate by gradual relaxation of the intercostal muscles. The volume of air inhaled or expelled is the tidal volume; the rhythmical inspiration and expiration at rest is tidal respiration. The stimuli of other mechanisms, e.g. exercise, which generate a need for more oxygen and a greater elimination of carbon dioxide, convert inspiration and expiration into more active processes, which may also recruit additional muscle power from accessory muscles, e.g. sternomastoid.

Internationally agreed physiological symbols

Descriptive

O_2	oxygen
N	nitrogen
CO_2	carbon dioxide
H_2O	water

Primary

C	concentration in blood phase
F	fractional concentration of gas in dry phase
P	gas pressure
P	partial pressure of gas
Q	blood flow (Q volume flow of blood)
R	respiratory quotient
V	gas volume

Descriptive/secondary
  Gas
  A   alveolar gas
  B   barometric
  D   dead space gas
  E   expired gas
  I   inspired gas

  Blood
  a   arterial
  c   pulmonary capillary
  v   venous

Definitive
  ·   denotes time
  –   denotes a mean value

Important examples of symbols
  F_{IO_2} fractional inspired concentration of oxygen
         (i.e. 0.2l in air at sea level)
  P_{AO_2} alveolar partial pressure of oxygen
  P_{aO_2} arterial partial pressure of oxygen
  V_d/V_t dead space to tidal volume ratio
  Q_s/Q_t shunt fraction
  C_{vO_2} mixed venous oxygen concentration
  R = V_{CO_2}/V_{O_2}

Evaluation of respiratory function

Tests can range from simple to complex, depending on the technology available. In clinical practice it is practical to use the simple ones about which there is now a sufficient bibliography.

Measurement of forced expiration

Forced expiratory manoeuvres are widely used because the measuring apparatus is cheap and convenient, and measurements are easy to make and reproducible. A variety of devices (e.g. peak flow meters, respirometers, wet and dry spirometers) is available for assessing expiratory manoeuvres, notably forced ones involving effort. Serial measurements, with patients as their own controls, give valuable information of the progress in pulmonary pathology. Results are non-specific, being indices that reflect combinations of a variety of physiological processes that include neuromuscular co-ordination, muscular power, pulmonary and chest wall compliance and patency of airways. They should never be used in isolation; merely as guides and indicators. Commonly used parameters are:

Forced expired volume in 1 second (FEV₁)

The volume of gas forcibly expired in 1 second. Usually extrapolated from a graph of a single forced expiratory manoeuvre and which is differentiated for volume and time. Normal value is 80% of the vital capacity in 1 second.

Forced vital capacity (FVC)

The maximum volume of gas forcefully expired after a deep inspiration. Usually measured in relation to FEV_1. The ratio is compared with nomograms for age, sex and height. The ratio of FEV_1:FVC can distinguish those with disease affecting conducting airways and with difficulty emptying their lungs, e.g. asthma, chronic bronchitis (low FEV_1 relative to FVC – obstructive) and those with both reduced commensurately, e.g. structural deformities, pulmonary oedema (low FEV_1 and lower than predicted FVC – restrictive).

Maximal breathing capacity (MBC)

The maximum volume of gas that can be breathed in 1 minute. Usually measured over a 15 s period. Average normal value is 120 litres per minute.

Peak expiratory flow rate (PEFR)

Measured either by a peak flow meter or off a forced spirometric trace, where it is the steepest part of the slope of volume expelled against time. It should be four to five times the MBC.

Pulmonary volumes and plethysmography

Some of the values can be acquired with the simple measuring devices mentioned above but for a complete set of the recognised compartmental divisions (four capacities and four volumes) it is necessary to measure the amount of air retained in the lungs at the end of maximum expiration – the residual volume (RV) – by whole body plethysmography. Similar caveats as those for forced expiratory manoeuvres apply to relevance and interpretation. The important derivatives from plethysmographic studies are:

Tidal volume (TV or Vt)

The volume of gas inspired or expired during normal, quiet ventilation. The normal value is generally 5 ml/kg body weight.

Total lung capacity (TLC)

The amount of gas in the lungs at the end of maximum inspiration, equal to:

inspiratory reserve volume (IRV) + TV + expiratory reserve volume (ERV) + RV

Vital capacity (VC)

Measured following maximal inspiration it represents the volume of gas that can forcefully be expired and is equal to:

IRV + TV + ERV

Inspiratory capacity (IC)

The volume of gas that can be inspired from the resting expiratory level, equal to:

IRV + TV

Functional residual capacity (FRC)

The volume of gas still in the lungs at the end of normal tidal ventilation, equal to:

ERV + RV

It is an important conceptual value as it represents the gaseous reservoir for oxygen during the majority of a respiratory cycle. Its relation to the index and closing volume (see below), is recognised as important in the understanding of the pathogenesis of some causes of hypoxaemia.

Compliance

Two structures contribute to the elastic resistance to inspiration. These are the chest wall and the pulmonary parenchyma: their separate contributions can be measured independently. The change in volume per unit of pressure applied to the lungs is the compliance. Generally expressed as litre/cm water, a low value usually represents stiff lungs.

Airways resistance

Narrowing of airways, small and large, creates a resistance to ventilation. An assessment of the contribution these may have to the work of breathing can be made from plethysmographic studies.

Marker-gas studies

Some important evaluative indices can be obtained by studies involving the inhalation of a variety of non-physiological substances. Relevant ones include:

Closing volume

The volume of gas in the lungs at the point when closure of airways is detected. Detected by study of the exhalation curves of marker gases such as helium, argon or nitrogen; a sudden steep inflection is believed to mark the onset of collapse of small basal airways, at which juncture their dependent alveoli begin to develop a V/Q ratio < 1 which contributes to physiological shunting.

Transfer factor

Carbon monoxide functions as a marker for gauging the transfer of oxygen from alveolus to pulmonary capillary. The concept of alveolar–capillary block has less credence nowadays as a major reason for any increase in A–a gradients, though it probably is relevant, in part, to the development of hypoxaemia in some cases of pulmonary fibrosis or pulmonary oedema.

Ventilation–perfusion scanning

Inhaled and injected radioactive markers such as technetium can be used to assess the matching of ventilation and perfusion in large areas of the lung. The results are of great value in the diagnosis of pulmonary emboli and in the assessment of fitness for pulmonary surgery.

Exercise testing

The study of exercise tolerance remains an important part of the assessment of patients with pulmonary disease. Oxygen uptake, carbon dioxide output, heart rate, respiratory rate and tidal volume are measured while patients undergo graduated exercise on treadmills or bicycle ergometers.

Tables of normal values
Table 4.1 Respiratory indices (adult 60–70 kg)

Weight of lung	800 g
Number of alveoli	296×10^6
Pulmonary capillary flow	5400 ml/min
Pulmonary capillary volume	60 ml
Respiratory rate	12–14/min
Dead space	150 ml (2.2 ml/kg)
Alveolar ventilation	4.2 litres/min
Tidal volume	400–600 ml
Minute volume	5–6 litres/min
Total pulmonary capacity	5.0–6.5 litres
Inspiratory reserve volume	3.30–3.75 litres
Expiratory reserve volume	0.95–1.20 litres
Functional residual capacity	2.3–2.8 litres
Residual volume	1.2–1.7 litres
Inspiratory capacity	3.6–4.3 litres
Vital capacity	4.2–4.8 litres
Forced expiratory volume in 1 s (FEV_1)	75% of VC
Peak expiratory flow rate	400 litres/min
Peak inspiratory flow rate	300 litres/min
Maximum ventilatory volume	120 litres/min
CO_2 diffusing capacity	17-20 ml/min/mmHg
Total compliance of lung and chest wall	0.1 litres/cm H_2O
Compliance of chest wall	0.2 litres/cm H_2O

Table 4.2 Gases (at BP 760 mmHg or 101.1 kPa)

Inspired air	
P_{O_2}	158 mmHg or 21.06 kPa
P_{CO_2}	0.3 mmHg or 0.04 kPa
P_{N_2}	596 mmHg or 79.46 kPa
P_{H_2O}	5 mmHg or 0.67 kPa
Expired air	
P_{O_2}	116 mmHg or 15.47 kPa
P_{CO_2}	28 mmHg or 3.73 kPa
P_{N_2}	568 mmHg or 75.73 kPa
P_{H_2O}	47 mmHg or 6.27 kPa
Alveolar gas	
P_{AO_2}	103 mmHg or 13.73 kPa
P_{ACO_2}	40 mmHg or 5.33 kPa
P_{AN_2}	570 mmHg or 75.99 kPa
P_{AH_2O}	47 mmHg or 6.27 kPa
Mixed venous blood	
P_{vO_2}	37–42 mmHg or 4.93–5.60 kPa
P_{vCO_2}	40–52 mmHg or 5.33–6.93 kPa
P_{vN_2}	573 mmHg or 76.39 kPa
pH	7.32–7.42
Arterial blood	
P_{aO_2}	90–110 mmHg or 12.00–14.67 kPa
P_{aCO_2}	34–46 mmHg or 4.53–6.13 kPa
P_{aN_2}	573 mmHg or 76.39 kPa
pH	7.36–7.44

Thoracocentesis

In intensive care this may be diagnostic or therapeutic. Posteroanterior and lateral X-rays should be obtained before the procedure, although in ventilated patients this is usually very difficult. With the patient sitting as upright as possible, the site of aspiration should be selected by X-ray. The skin and soft tissues are then infiltrated with local anaesthetic, which is also injected around the periostium, followed by aspiration of the pleural cavity just above the rib. With the definitive cannula the pleural space is reached in the same place with gentle aspiration and the needle removed. A three-way tap is attached to the cannula and the fluid aspirated progressively. Remember that sudden drainage of large pleural effusions may cause re-expansion pulmonary oedema.

As the lung re-expands the patient coughs. After the aspiration is finished, a new control radiograph is obtained.

The minimal equipment for thoracocentesis is:

- 50 ml plastic syringe
- large plastic cannula with attached needle
- N 15 blade
- plastic three-way tap
- gauze swabs.

Pleural drainage

An indwelling underwater-seal tube may be required in treating pneumothorax, draining blood, fluid or pus.

Lie the patient in bed propped up at 60° with pillows, lying with the affected side uppermost and the arm placed behind the head to expose the axilla. Prepare the chest wall. The best site for a tube for pneumothorax is high up in the axilla, third or fourth space, mid-axillary line, just lateral to pectoralis major. Here it is unobtrusive and comfortable. A minimal amount of muscle is encountered. Older textbooks recommend the second space, mid-clavicular line, but this practice should be a last resort, as pectoralis major is a bulky muscle, the internal mammary may be damaged and in females the scar is unsightly.

Fluid should be drained through a lower point – the seventh or eighth space, mid-axillary line. Remember this is just above the diaphragm. Proceed with extreme caution and ensure fluid is readily aspirated with a 21 G needle before proceeding. If in doubt ask for an ultrasound or insert Lipiodol under X-ray screening, or go a space higher.

Care is taken in making the skin incision small enough to ensure a tight fit. The traditional purse-string is unnecessary unless a leak occurs around the tube. Either a Malécot tube or Argyle catheter may be used. When apical placement is desired, the latter is preferred. Make sure the outermost hole is within the pleural space to avoid surgical emphysema. Secure the tube with a strong ligature and strapping.

Removal of tube

This is surprisingly simple. Place the patient in position as above. Drapes and gowns are unnecessary, but gloves must be worn. Remove dressings and retaining stitch. Ask the patient to take a deep breath *in*, to expand the lung right up to chest wall, and to hold the breath against a closed glottis – now pull out the tube in a single firm action and close the two edges of the incision with the fingers of the left hand. A single deep suture can now be placed to close, or a stitch, left *in situ* when the tube is inserted initially, can be tied.

Mediastinoscopy

Mediastinoscopy is performed for establishment of histology where enlarged mediastinal glands are found by X-rays or CT scans. The incision is made midway between the bottom of the sternal notch and the cricoid cartilage. Scissor dissection is made through the pre-tracheal fascia and then the finger is passed behind this fascial plane in front of the trachea.

The mediastinoscope can follow this track, examining all tissues on the way. if there is any doubt before biopsy, a presumed lymph node can be distinguished from a vessel by prior needle aspiration.

Anterior mediastinoscopy

Glands around the aortic arch to the left of the tracheal bifurcation are not accessible to mediastinoscopy. Similarly, anterior mediastinal glands on either side require a more anterior approach. An incision of 6–10 cm is made over the second cartilage, which is resected subperichondrially and the internal mammary artery divided after ligation. The pleura can then frequently be swept laterally without penetration, giving access to the mediastinum.

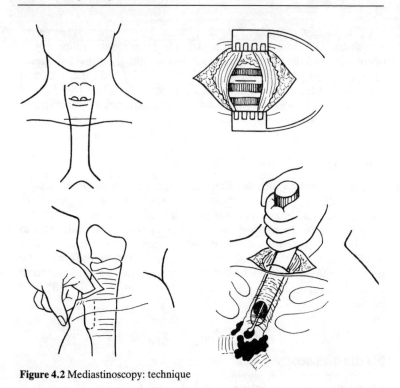

Figure 4.2 Mediastinoscopy: technique

Careful haemostasis and avoidance of phrenic nerves are important.

Biopsy of lung

Lung biopsy can be bronchial, transtracheal, fine-needle, Trucut and open.

Modern fibreoptic instruments permit very peripheral lung tissue to be biopsied transbronchially.

Fine-needle biopsy has made accessible for histology peripheral lesions beyond the reach of bronchoscopy, such as localised infection in children and in immunocompromised patients, inoperable lesions and lesions in the apex.

Tomograms and multiplane screening facilities are necessary. Contraindications include bleeding tendency, multiple emphysematous bullae with poor pulmonary function, and circumstances liable to provoke pneumothorax, haemoptysis or air embolus.

Open lung biopsy may be necessary when transbronchial or percutaneous methods have failed. An adequate mini-thoracotomy over the most suspicious area is followed by a mini-wedge-resection, using a stapler if possible. Avoid the temptation to lop off the lingula just because it is easy; always remove the most pathological piece. Routine closure with underwater drainage is carried out, as for a full thoracotomy.

A half-way house which is underused is the thoracoscopy, especially useful for pleural or very peripheral lesions, and more applicable with modern fibreoptic endoscopes. The endoscope is introduced through one trochar cannula and the biopsy forceps through another. Biopsies are then taken under direct vision, and of course a drain is finally inserted through one of the cannulae.

Endotracheal intubation

Every doctor should be adept in this as, apart from general anaesthesia and mechanical ventilation, it may be necessary for removal of aspirated material, airway obstruction or trauma, and similar life-threatening conditions.

A curved laryngoscope (McIntosh), which goes into the vallecula, is more common than a straight one (Miller), which goes behind the epiglottis. The tube size in general is 2–4 for infants, 4–7 for children and 7–10 for adults. The laryngoscope should display the vocal chords and the tube inserted through them under direct vision. Laryngeal trauma, oesophageal intubation and overinflation of the cuff, with subsequent mucosal damage and stenosis, should be avoided.

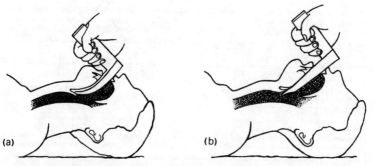

(a)   (b)

Figure 4.3 Endotracheal intubation with (a) a curved McIntosh laryngoscope and (b) a straight Miller laryngoscope

Cricothyroidotomy

This includes the 'mini-tracheostomy'. A small cannula is introduced through the cricothyroid membrane as an emergency for acute obstruction with difficult intubation, or electively for removal of sputum where tracheostomy is not thought to be necessary. Through this cannula secretions can be aspirated, oxygen administered, the bronchi washed and nebulised drugs given.

Patients known to have difficulty with sputum clearance, bad left ventricular function, larygneal incoordination, or poor mental co-operation are potential candidates for this procedure.

If a proper tracheostomy is to be done, the mini-tracheostomy should not be employed. Of course, low tracheal obstruction is not helped by it.

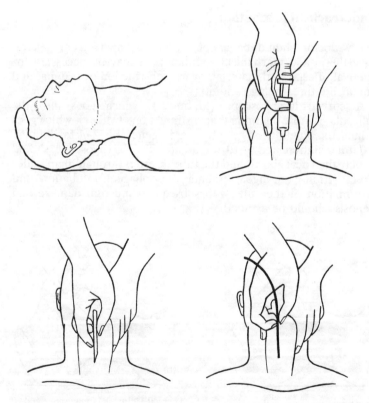

Figure 4.4 Mini-tracheostomy: technique

Tracheostomy

May be urgent (occlusion of the upper airway by trauma or diphtheria) or elective (in cases of prolonged intubation for ventilation or other purposes). The procedure is as for mediastinoscopy, making an incision midway between cricoid cartilage and the bottom of the sternal notch, followed by scissor dissection of pretracheal fascia and the anterior surface of the trachea itself. Through the second and third ring the incision is made and it can be horizontal, vertical, inverted U-shape or X-shaped.

The most important aspect is the care of the tube: bronchial aspiration hourly; change of dressing daily; change of tube weekly.

Complications

- operative bleeding
- pneumothorax
- tracheo-oesophageal fistula
- laryngeal nerve injury
- paratracheal intubation
- obstruction of the tube
- aspiration
- infection
- tracheo-arterial fistula
- stenosis
- tracheomalacia
- granuloma
- permanent stoma.

The pressure in the cuff should be just sufficient to prevent excessive leakage from the ventilation circuit. High pressures may cause mucosal destruction with subsequent erosion and stricture.

Bronchoscopy

Rigid

1. *Diagnostic*: mainly to identify tumours, sites of haemoptysis, stenosis or rupture.
2. *Therapeutic*: for removal of foreign body, retained secretions, obstructing plugs, laser resection of malignant obstructions, trauma to airways, blockage of bronchus, in severe haemoptysis or fistula.

Generally, rigid bronchoscopy is performed under general anaesthesia. Staff should be aware of abnormal coagulation and electrocardiographic or radiological hazards. The patient should be starving and premedicated with atropine (0.6–1.2 mg i.v. or i.m.).

Heavy bleeding may be controlled with a swab soaked in adrenaline, applied for 2–3 minutes. Massive bleeding may be treated by pressure with a swab, Fogarty catheter or Thompson bronchial blocker, fluid replacement, and in some cases, thoracotomy.

Fibreoptic

A mainly diagnostic procedure providing a good view of all subsegmental bronchi. Bronchoalveolar lavage, bronchial brushings, bronchial biopsies and transbronchial lung biopsies (TBLB) may be taken.

Fibreoptic bronchoscopy is performed under local anaesthetic. Its disadvantage is that it cannot cope with a large loss of blood. It is usually not suitable for the removal of a foreign body.

Important tests

1. Spirometry: FEV_1, VC. If $FEV_1 < 1$ litre, do arterial blood gas (use supplemental oxygen at bronchoscopy).
2. ECG.
3. Chest X-ray: PA and lateral.
4. Platelets and prothrombin time before TBLB.

Preparation

1. Consent form.
2. Starve for at least 4 hours.
3. Premedication: 0.6 mg atropine i.m. to dry secretions.
4. Sedation is achieved with benzodiazepines (Diazemuls 10 mg) or Omnopon 10–20 mg or both.

Acute respiratory failure

Definition

Respiratory failure is defined in terms of function, *not* in terms of arbitrary mechanics. Thus, arterial blood gas analysis is essential for diagnosis. There are two accepted types of respiratory failure:

Type I. Arterial Po_2 less than 8.0 kPa, whilst breathing air; also termed *hypoxaemic failure.*

Type II. Pao_2 criteria as type I, plus arterial Pco_2 greater than 6.5 kPa; also termed *ventilatory* failure.

Note: hypoxaemia is *always* present and essential for diagnosis.

Aetiology

There is considerable overlap in the disease associated with types I and II respiratory failure, and hypoxaemic failure often leads to ventilatory failure with progression of the underlying disease. However, the pattern of failure does vary with the basic disease process.

Type I

Hypoxaemic failure alone is usually associated with diseases of the pulmonary parenchyma, interstitium or alveoli, for example:

- lobar or bronchopneumonia
- pulmonary oedema
- asthma
- chronic obstructive airways disease
- pulmonary infiltration (e.g. carcinomatosis, fungi, etc.)
- adult respiratory distress syndrome, etc.

Type II

All diseases that produce hypoxaemic failure may progress to ventilatory failure in later stages, but hypercapnia occuring early in the clinical course is seen with a different group of diseases:

1. Diseases affecting the CNS:
   - drugs, e.g. opiates
   - trauma
   - coma, whatever the aetiology
   - brain stem disease, such as tumours or infarcts.
2. Neuromuscular diseases:
   - Guillain–Barré syndrome
   - poliomyelitis
   - myaesthenia gravis
   - tetanus.
3. Diseases affecting the thoracic cage:
   - trauma, usually severe with large flail segments

- kyphoscoliosis
- obesity.

This list is not comprehensive and is given to illustrate the different pattern of disease only. The distinction is important mainly for guidance in management (see below).

Pathophysiology

Hypoxaemia is virtually always due to ventilation–perfusion (V/Q) imbalance within the lungs. True diffusion block occurs only in rare diseases such as alveolar proteinosis, and the vast majority of clinical conditions associated with hypoxia produce this by mismatching of ventilation and pulmonary blood flow, usually in a non-uniform manner. The resultant V/Q mismatch produces marked intrapulmonary *shunting* of blood.

Hypercapnia is due either to severe, diffuse pulmonary disease, such that there is insufficient functioning lung left to cope with the rate of production of CO_2, or to an interference with the mechanics of delivery of gas to the alveolus, as is seen with, for example, central respiratory depression by drugs. These circumstances also produce *V/Q* mismatching, but of a different type to that seen with Type I failure, resulting in *increase in physiological dead-space*.

Effects of respiratory failure

Irrespective of the underlying disease, the physiological abnormalities seen with the onset of respiratory failure will produce secondary effects on the body. These effects vary both with the severity of the physiological disturbance and its duration, and predominantly involve the cardiorespiratory systems.

Hypoxia

1. *Respiratory effects.* The principal effect of hypoxia is to stimulate ventilation, mainly by stimulating the peripheral chemoreceptors found in the region of the carotid body. The resulting increase in ventilation is, however, limited by the associated fall in the PaCO_2, which will in turn depress ventilation by a central effect on the respiratory centre in the brain stem. The usual finding, therefore, in type I respiratory failure, is hypoxia plus modest hypocapnia (1–1.5 kPa below normal).

2. *Cardiovascular effects.* There are variable effects of hypoxia on different vascular beds, and the common findings are:
   (a) Increase in blood pressure, cardiac output, and peripheral resistance. At a later stage with increasing hypoxia, these indices fall.
   (b) Vasoconstriction in the skin and general visceral circulations, including the kidney.
   (c) Dilatation of the cerebral and coronary circulations.
   (d) Increase in pulmonary blood flow, associated with an increase in both pulmonary vascular resistance and pulmonary arterial pressure. These changes, if chronic, result in permanent pulmonary vascular changes and lead to cor pulmonale.
3. *Metabolic effects.* Hypoxia of sufficient severity or duration will lead to alteration of cellular metabolism. This will result in the production of various fixed acids, normally excreted by the kidneys. The buffering capacity of the extracellular fluid is limited, as is the rate of excretion by the kidneys, and hypoxia is often associated with a significant non-respiratory (also termed metabolic) acidosis.
4. *Effects on bone marrow.* Chronic hypoxia results in an increase in production of erythropoietin by the kidney. This will cause an increase in red blood cell mass, the resultant secondary polycythaemia being distinguished from primary polycythaemia rubra vera by not affecting the white blood cell or platelet counts. This effect is not seen in acute hypoxia.

Hypercapnia

1. *Respiratory effects.* As $Paco_2$ rises, there is an increase in tidal and minute volumes and respiratory rate, due to a direct stimulation of the respiratory centre. However, as the CO_2 level rises, eventually the effect changes to a global depression of CNS activity, including the respiratory centre. This is seen with $Paco_2$ levels in excess of 12 kPa and is associated with depressed consciousness and coma.
2. *Cardiovascular effects.* As with hypoxia, hypercapnia produces differing effects on different vascular beds:
   (a) constriction of visceral vascular beds, including kidney;
   (b) dilatation of the vascular beds of skin, brain, and heart;
   (c) increase of cardiac output.

A particular concern with the combination of hypoxia and hypercapnia, as can be seen from the above effects, is their additive effect on the kidney, both resulting in renal vasoconstriction and thereby producing considerable risk of renal failure.

Clinical assessment

Assessment of a patient in respiratory failure is essentially clinical, in particular the decisions relating to treatment, especially active intervention such as intubation and artificial ventilation; the following aspects must all be taken into account:

1. Clinical features of the underlying disease, if any.
2. Presence or absence of breathlessness/dyspnoea.
3. Strength of cough and ability to clear secretions.
4. Quantity and nature of sputum.
5. Breathing patterns: increased or decreased respiratory efforts, the presence of abdominal distention, paradoxical movements, obesity interfering with respiration, and, most important, the characteristic breathing pattern associated with fatigue.
6. Measurements of respiratory mechanics are of limited value in the acute situation and trends in simple bedside observations are of more value. Those of most value are respiratory frequency, minute volume and chest wall movement. More complicated measures, such as FEV_1 or PEF, require full co-operation and have little part to play in the patient with acute respiratory failure.
7. Clinical features of abnormal gas exchange, as described above, may be present, remembering that cyanosis is only present if there is at least 5 g of reduced haemoglobin in the blood, and this will only occur if blood with a normal haemoglobin level is less than 75% saturated (representing a Pao_2 of less than 5.3 kPa).
8. Arterial blood gas analysis is essential. Most value is obtained from serial measurements and trends over periods of time or with therapy. However, decisions about whether to ventilate or not are usually taken in conjunction with the patient's clinical condition.
9. Chest X-ray, especially if previous radiographs are available for comparison.
10. Most important, the *past history*. Many patients present in established failure and an accurate history may be the only way to spot those patients with underlying chronic disease.

Treatment

Added inspired, humidified oxygen is essential. Inotropes, afterload reducers and diuretics may be necessary for the treatment of pulmonary oedema. Bronchodilators are useful for those with evidence of reversible airways obstruction. Physiotherapy may help to loosen and clear retained sputum and re-expand collapsed lungs. For those whose major difficulty is failure to clear large airway secretions, the use of cricothyroid membrane puncture with a small bore mini-tracheostomy is recommended.

Positive pressure ventilation

Failure of first-line measures, progressive deterioration, and exhaustion are indications for positive pressure ventilation. The type of ventilator and pattern of ventilation depend on clinical indications. Conventional techniques are usually suitable. High-frequency ventilation techniques have been advocated for conditions where a raised mean intrathoracic pressure is to be avoided, e.g. bronchopleural fistula. There is some evidence that these techniques are also more effective in type II respiratory failure than conventional positive pressure ventilation. Wide pathological discrepancies between an individual's lungs indicate double lumen tracheal intubation for differential ventilation of the individual lungs.

Adult respiratory distress syndrome

Definition

'Acute respiratory failure associated with non-respiratory sepsis or trauma'.

The definition of adult respiratory distress syndrome (ARDS) unfortunately varies considerably and many clinicians apply the term to any disease resulting in the association of increasing A–a gradient and diffuse pulmonary infiltration on chest X-ray, in the absence of left heart failure. This definition is too wide, and includes direct thoracic trauma, aspiration pneumonia, and even viral pneumonias, enabling the term to be applied indiscriminately, undermining the value of the diagnosis.

The term ARDS is restricted in this discussion to primary non-respiratory pathology (thereby eliminating those diseases such as primary pneumonias), in which respiratory failure ensues as a secondary complication.

Aetiology

The principal associations of ARDS are septicaemia and non-thoracic trauma. Some would include thoracic trauma, pneumonias and primary intrathoracic diseases as causes of ARDS, but this decreases the usefulness of the term. Many pulmonary diseases have a common final pathway of pathophysiology and similar end-stage microscopic changes – the lung can respond to injury of any type in a restricted way.

The syndrome was originally recognised following non-thoracic trauma and the most common association seen in most intensive care units is related to sepsis, usually intra-abdominal. The development of ARDS is independent of the actual site of trauma or of the nature of the infecting organism.

The exact mechanism underlying ARDS is still to be elucidated. With sepsis as the aetiological agent, endotoxin released from bacteria initiates numerous events at the cellular level, involving activation of systems such as the prostaglandins, kinins and histamine. Clotting and complement cascades are activated, with liberation of substances which damage the pulmonary endothelium. White blood cells are held in the pulmonary microcirculation and there is local release, from platelets in particular, of the various prostaglandins; endothelial interaction results in the generation of free radicals of oxygen, which in turn will produce further pulmonary cellular damage.

Total pulmonary water and capillary permeability increase and the normal microvascular control alters, with areas of hypoxia and maldistribution of blood to the lungs.

Clinical features

The principal features are dyspnoea, fall in Pao_2, and the development of diffuse pulmonary opacities on chest X-ray. The underlying illness may overshadow the insidious changes of ARDS.

Dyspnoea in a patient with peripheral or abdominal trauma or sepsis may be caused by the underlying illness, for which he may already be artificially ventilated. In these circumstances, arterial gas monitoring becomes mandatory. A low Pao_2 may be the first sign of development of ARDS; this may be associated with the primary disease without ARDS and the important finding is a progressive fall. The only other clinical finding, besides dyspnoea, is the development of diffuse crepitations. Sputum production in ARDS is minimal.

Chest X-ray after abdominal trauma or sepsis commonly shows basal collapse and consolidation. This is the likeliest cause of hypoxia in these circumstances and ARDS should only be considered if diffuse alveolar shadowing develops. The X-ray appearance is similar to diffuse bronchopneumonia, acute pulmonary oedema and all other causes of diffuse alveolar shadowing.

Treatment

Treatment is based on the same principles as those of a patient in respiratory failure, whatever the cause (see p. 218). Specific therapy for ARDS is not available at present as the basic underlying pathophysiology is not yet known.

Theoretically, specific treatment is with:

1. *Steroids.* Experiments have shown reduction in mortality with steroids administered early in the clinical course, often before the insult. In reality, steroids are counterproductive and a major clinical trial was abandoned.
2. *Prostaglandin E_1 (PGE$_1$).* No difference in mortality rates has been found.
3. *Sequential haemofiltration.* This may remove endotoxins; research is in progress.

Mechanical ventilation (see also p. 65)

Indications

Elective

Mainly postoperative ventilation, with increasingly sick patients and complex surgical procedures.

Postoperative ventilation is more often chosen for:

1. Ensuring satisfactory oxygenation, a particular concern in the post-abdominal surgery patient.
2. Full control of P_{CO_2} level, allowing better control of acid–base balance.
3. Allowing analgesia to be administered until the patient is completely pain-free, without concern about concomitant respiratory depression.
4. Allowing extensive tracheobronchial toilet and preventing postoperative atelactasis (not substantial).
5. Other aspects of postoperative care and resuscitation, such as fluid and electrolyte balance, can be looked after without ventilatory concerns.

Treatment of respiratory failure

Irrespective of the aetiology of respiratory failure, intubation and artificial ventilation may be required in the more severe cases (see p. 223). The decision as to when to intervene is often very difficult and depends on many factors:

1. Serial blood gas results, with deteriorating Pao_2 and rising $Paco_2$. The onset of ventilatory failure is often the critical point in the clinical course, especially in acute illnesses without underlying pulmonary disease.
2. Ability to clear secretions, a factor linked to (3).
3. Fatigue, which is often the critical factor in precipitating intervention, and although everyone can recognise a patient who is fatigued, it is difficult to define precisely. The onset of fatigue in acute respiratory failure often coincides with the onset of ventilatory failure, with rising $Paco_2$, decreased ability to expectorate, diminished respiratory effort and often a decreased conscious level.

Types of artificial ventilation

Two basic approaches to artificial ventilation are recognised: the use of negative or positive pressure devices.

Negative pressure devices

Tank or cuirass ventilators exert a negative pressure around the outside of the patient's thorax, expanding the chest and sucking air into the lungs via the patient's normal airway, thus mimicking normal respiratory mechanics. These devices are rarely used in acute illness but are mainly used in patients with chronic disease, when long-term home ventilation is necessary. They are not considered further here.

Positive pressure devices

These deliver a positive pressure to the patient's airway and force gas down the normal respiratory passages. Intubation of the trachea is essential in some form. The apparatus is more efficient and more manoeuvrable than that for negative pressure and allows access to the patient. Positive pressure ventilators have now developed to a highly sophisticated level, enabling us to manipulate respiratory mechanics and question accepted concepts of respiratory physiology.

Objectives of intermittent positive pressure ventilation (IPPV)

1. Improved distribution of gases in the lung. This will improve V/Q imbalance, leading to an increase in Pao_2.
2. Accurate control of Fio_2, not possible with face masks, especially in a patient who is confused or disorientated because of respiratory failure.
3. Reduction in consumption of oxygen. Respiratory failure increases the work of breathing, on occasion to as high as 20% of the total oxygen consumption. In a patient who has difficulty in oxygenation due to the underlying disease, eliminating work of breathing can have a significant effect.
4. Control of Pco_2 level. With severe disease it may not always be possible to reduce the $Paco_2$ to normal but it is usually possible to bring this level down to a safe range, i.e. below 9–10 kPa.
5. Enables effective tracheal toilet and physiotherapy, perhaps one of the most important aspects of respiratory care. Also allows sampling of sputum for accurate diagnosis.
6. Other benefits include allowing complete pain control and relief of distress, as discussed above.

Adverse effects of IPPV

Circulatory effects
The use of positive pressure ventilation means that at no time during the respiratory cycle does the intrathoracic pressure become subatmospheric. Thus the normal effect of the 'thoracic pump', enhancing venous return to the right side of the heart, is lost. In addition, we are imposing a high mean intrathoracic pressure and so impeding venous return. In patients with normal circulating blood volume and intact cardiovascular system reflexes, adjustment occurs fairly rapidly, with minimal effect on cardiac output. However, in a patient who is dehydrated or with a diminished circulating volume, or with impaired ability to compensate, IPPV can result in a marked fall in cardiac output and blood pressure, necessitating vigorous resuscitation.

Respiratory effects
A positive intrathoracic pressure has been shown to produce altered capillary blood flow, so that on occasions initiation of IPPV may produce a fall in Pao_2, due to an increase in shunting, overshadowing the beneficial effect of improved distribution of ventilation. This is more likely to occur with IPPV in a patient with normal lungs and, in practice, in respiratory failure the beneficial

effects outweigh the adverse effects, with an improvement in oxygenation, not a deterioration.

Of more concern is the possibility of barotrauma to the lungs. The use of high inflating pressures has been shown to produce mechanical damage to the pulmonary parenchyma, at its worst resulting in a pneumothorax which would rapidly progress to tension and myocardial tamponade. Short of pulmonary disruption, pathological changes such as bronchiolectasis have been reported. The significance of these findings is uncertain and it is not known whether full resolution occurs with time. Also uncertain is the contribution of barotrauma to the development of pulmonary fibrosis following prolonged IPPV with high oxygen concentrations, so-called 'oxygen toxicity'.

Acid–base balance

Control of P_{CO_2} levels allows regulation of one component of overall acid–base balance. However, reduction of a chronically elevated P_{CO_2} will produce a metabolic alkalosis until the kidneys can compensate. Also, rapid falls in P_{CO_2} will have an adverse effect on both cerebral blood flow and cardiac output, since a rise in CO_2 level increases cerebral blood flow directly, and enhances cardiac output secondary to an increase in sympathetic activity. Also reported are significant shifts in potassium distribution between intra- and extracellular spaces following rapid falls in P_{CO_2} levels, on occasion producing ventricular fibrillation. Chronically elevated levels of P_{CO_2} must be reduced slowly and with caution.

Other effects

Many other, more minor effects are seen, perhaps the most common being an increase in antidiuretic hormone (ADH) levels. This may contribute to the diuresis commonly seen when IPPV is discontinued.

Glossary

Types of ventilators

- Flow generator
- Pressure generator
- Minute volume divider
- Volume controlled
- Pressure controlled

Basic controls

- Minute volume
- Tidal volume
- Rate
- I:E ratio

Ancillary settings

- PEEP (positive end expiratory pressure)
- CPAP (continuous positive airway pressure)
- IMV (intermediate mandatory ventilation)
- SIMV (synchronous IMV)
- MMV (mandatory minute ventilation)
- Trigger
- Pressure support
- HFV (high frequency ventilation)
- Jet ventilation

Emergencies during IPPV

Potentially fatal events are not common in a modern ITU, provided adequate levels of staff are available and appropriate monitoring is carried out. Should either be unavailable, then the risk associated with IPPV is unacceptable, and should a catastrophe occur, the unit would be medicolegally culpable. The single most important requirement is trained nursing staff.

Machine-related emergencies

Power-failure

Units with electrically driven ventilators should always have an emergency back-up generator, often with a secondary back-up link to other generators within the hospital. Should failure occur, automatic switching to the back-up supply will occur within seconds. Only in the rare instance of failure of the back-up link should a grid power failure pose a threat.

Action: Immediate disconnection from the ventilator circuit and hand ventilation via a Water's circuit or Ambu bag with 100% oxygen.

Oxygen supply failure

It would be extremely rare for a central supply to fail. Problems with the pipelines between reservoir and wall outlets do occur but, again, are rare. The most common failure is at the wall outlet itself, usually the fitting of the Schroeder valve into the socket. (It may appear to be connected!) Once the valve is fixed correctly, the common sites for supply failure are any junctions in the circuit from valve to ventilator.

Inspired oxygen concentrations must be monitored continuously, despite the rarity of mainline supply failure, since an unrecognised fall in delivered oxygen will rapidly lead to cerebral hypoxic damage. Also mandatory is an alarm system, both auditory and visual, should failure occur.

Action: Immediate disconnection from the ventilator and hand ventilation via an alternative circuit as above, with 100% oxygen. An alternative supply of oxygen must always be available at any site where artificial ventilation is carrried out, usually as bottled compressed oxygen.

Failure to deliver preset volumes (despite intact supply and intact patient-circuit)

Provided there is no leak between ventilator and patient (see below), this always means a leak in the internal circuit of the ventilator. Mechanically-driven ventilators, such as the Cape, often leak at the bellows, whilst electronically-controlled ventilators, such as the Servo 900 series, have weak interfaces between the various transducers or sensors within the control box. A serious, but rarely critical, deficiency in the volumes of delivered gases may occur. In a patient who requires a high inspired oxygen concentration, a small fall in delivered volume may again produce rapid hypoxia.

Because the volume of gas actually delivered to the patient is the vital consideration, it is essential to measure the patient's *expired* tidal and minute volumes. Also, it is essential to have an audible and visual alarm system, adjustable so that small falls in volumes of delivered gases can be detected.

Action: Immediate disconnection from the ventilator and hand ventilation with 100% oxygen as above. If there is any doubt about the ventilator, it must be replaced until fully checked.

Patient-circuit emergencies

Disconnection

In any patient-circuit, there may be more than eight or nine connections, each a potentially weak point. Minimising these will decrease the risk, and a disconnecting alarm minimises time between disconnection and recognition.

Action: If the site of disconnection is immediately obvious, rapid reconnection is all that is required. If it is not apparent where the disconnection has occurred, the patient must be hand ventilated, via an alternative circuit as above, with 100% oxygen until the situation has been rectified.

Leak within the circuit

A site that is particularly prone to leak gases from the circuit is the heated-water type humidifier, mainly at the junction where the water reservoir bowl screws on to the manifold. Leaks in the patient-circuit are probably more common than from the inside of the ventilator and are recognised by a significant discrepancy between the measured inspired and expired volumes. Although termed 'inspired volume', this measurement is actually the volume of gas delivered by the ventilator into the connecting circuit, whereas the 'expired volume' measures that breathed out by the patient, and is assumed to be the same as the true inspired volume.

The 'disconnect' alarm actually also acts to detect leaks occurring after ventilation has been started. This is because it relates to the patient's expired tidal or minute volume and is adjustable so as to be able to set at a level just below the patient's actual level of ventilation.

Action: As for Disconnection (above).

Cuff rupture

This usually occurs soon after placement of the endotracheal tube, probably as a result of damage during intubation, especially nasal intubation, but may occur at any time whilst a patient is intubated (also applies to tracheostomy tubes). The result is the same as with leaks at other sites in the patient-circuit and it is recognised by the development of an obvious loss of gas from the mouth of the patient during the inspiratory phase.

Action: Check first that the cuff has not been accidentally deflated, by emptying any residual air out of the cuff and reinflating with the same volume of air that was originally used. Once having confirmed that cuff rupture has occurred, the endotracheal or tracheostomy tube must be replaced. Provided that the patient is not becoming hypoxic there is usually time to organise all necessary personnel and equipment and carry out the procedure under controlled conditions. Occasionally, with severe pulmonary disorder, hypoxia ensues and replacement of the tube must be carried out immediately. Thus it is essential that at all times the equipment for intubation is readily available. Remember also that if a problem arises with a tracheostomy tube, especially soon after formation of the tracheal stoma, it may be quicker and safer to reintubate orally than to attempt tracheostomy tube changes.

Blockage of tracheal tube

This may arise with both endotracheal and tracheostomy tubes and is usually caused by inspissated sputum.

As these cuffs when inflated are 'floppy', so as to minimise the pressure exerted on the tracheal endothelium, the cuff can herniate over the lumen of the tube and cause partial or complete obstruction.

Blockage of the tube is recognised by a rise in inflating pressure without change in delivered tidal volume. The rise in inflating pressure may also be caused by obstruction in the circuit at other sites, for instance, the expiratory filter (see below). In this circumstance, a check of all such sites must be carried out in a routine order so that the cause can be rapidly identified.

Suggested check list:
1. Is patient's chest still moving? Has patient developed bronchospasm?
2. Disconnect from ventilator. Pressure still high: inspiratory circuit or ventilator problem.
3. Pressure falls to zero on disconnection. Attempt to pass suction catheter down tube. Will not pass: tube blocked.
4. Suction catheter passes: problem distal to tube. ?Pneumo-thorax.
5. No pneumothorax: problem in expiratory circuit. ?Expiratory filter blocked.
6. Expiratory filter not blocked: problem in ventilator.

Action: according to the defect found.

Patient emergencies

Pneumothorax

The development of a pneumothorax while the patient is being artificially ventilated is a real threat to life, since this can rapidly progress to tamponade. Resultant cardiovascular collapse may occur within minutes of pulmonary rupture as air is forced under positive pressure into the pleural space. A high index of suspicion is essential to be able to recognise this complication as early as possible and insert chest drains, if necessary without radiological confirmation.

Pneumothorax is more likely to occur in children during poorly-controlled hand ventilation and during the recovery phase of a severe, long illness, when high inflating pressures are still required but some areas of the lung are clearing.

Pulmonary embolism

The effect of pulmonary embolism is influenced by a series of factors: size of the embolus, number of emboli, time for embolisation, composition of emboli (firm with platelets, soft with fibrin) and the presence of pre-existent cardiopulmonary disease. The presentation may therefore be: sudden postoperative death in a patient making a normal recovery; cardiogenic shock; chest pain and dyspnoea; pleuritic pain with pyrexia and haemoptysis.

Post-mortem studies show that pulmonary embolism is found in 10–15% of patients dying in hospital. The important clinical clues are:

- sudden onset of dyspnoea
- pleuritic pain
- haemoptysis
- hypoxia
- elevated JVP and third heart sound
- clinical evidence of deep venous thrombosis
- predisposing factors: surgery, fractures, pregnancy, contraceptives, prolonged immbolisation.

The electrocardiogram may be normal. Nevertheless, it may show atrial fibrillation, right bundle branch block, T wave inversion in inferior and septal leads, and pattern of $S_1Q_3T_3$.

Chest X-rays may also be normal initially. Later, pleural effusion, wedge collapse and oligaemic lung may appear.

Echocardiogram shows right ventricular dilatation and elevated pulmonary arterial pressure.

Blood gases show hypoxia and low P_{CO_2}.

V/Q scan shows areas of perfusion defect with normal ventilation. Pulmonary angiography is the definitive investigation and the diagnostic gold standard.

Treatment of pulmonary embolism varies according to the clinical presentation. Oxygen and analgesia should be administered routinely.

Minor embolism requires heparin: 7500 U stat dose, followed by 35–40 000 U in 24 hours by constant-infusion pump. The KCCT or PTT should be checked after 4 hours and the infusion adjusted. Heparin has a half-life of 90 min, therefore, it is vital to maintain constant infusion. The aim is to keep KCCT or PT around two to three times control. If the patient is over-anticoagulated, the pump is switched off for 30 minutes.

Once the patient is stable, usually after 3–7 days, oral anticoagulants are started, taking into account that it takes at least 2 days for warfarin to become effective, so there is an overlap period.

Major life-threatening embolism should be investigated promptly with pulmonary angiography. The extent of the embolism should be determined, and if possible, the pulmonary arterial pressures recorded. Streptokinase 250 000 U loading dose followed by 100 000 U hourly i.v. infusion can be administered directly on to the clot via the angiography catheter. If effective, it is maintained for about 48 hours or until the right heart pressures drop, when the patient is reverted back to heparin.

If the condition does not improve rapidly, pulmonary embolectomy may be undertaken. Some technical points are worth mentioning:

1. Once the median sternotomy is completed, soft vascular clamps are applied to both cavae and the heart will empty in 5–6 beats;
2. The pulmonary artery is opened, the embolus scooped out, and the incision closed initially with a side biting clamp before releasing the clamps from the cavae.

Massive haemoptysis

This is arbitrarily defined as the expectoration of 600 ml of blood in a 24-hour period. Frequently the patient has compromised pulmonary function, which is further complicated by the risk of drowning in blood and by hypovolaemia.

Some important causes of massive haemoptysis are:

- lung cancer
- tuberculosis
- bronchiectasis
- lung abscess
- fungal disease
- aortic aneurysms
- general bleeding disorders
- trauma.

General measures in the management of this situation are:

1. *Resuscitation.* Insertion of a large bore i.v. cannula, cross-matching of blood, central venous pressure line, urinary catheter, fluid replacement.
2. *Conservative management.* Patient on bed-rest in upright position. Humidified oxygen by facemask. Broad spectrum antibiotics if the sputum is purulent until proper culture results are obtained.
3. *Investigations:*

   - full blood count
   - biochemistry
   - blood gases
   - clotting studies
   - chest X-rays
   - sputum for Gram staining, culture and cytology
   - flexible bronchoscopy.

If the bleeding persists, rigid bronchoscopy under general anaesthesia, in order to localise and contain the haemorrhage and to evacuate blood clots from within the remaining bronchial tree, is performed. Full preparations for emergency thoracotomy should be ready. Once the bronchoscope is inside the airways, the non-bleeding areas are selectively ventilated. Ice-cold saline lavage is then performed down the main bronchus of the bleeding lung, using 50 ml aliquots and ventilating the non-bleeding lung between instillation and aspiration.

If the procedure fails to stop the bleeding, balloon tamponade of the bleeding segmental bronchus (if possible) or occlusion of the proximal bronchus is attempted. Continuous haemorrhage is an indication for either an emergency bronchial arteriography and embolisation, or thoracotomy.

If no further massive bleeding occurs, the patient is stabilised for further medical or surgical treatment, according to the cause of bleeding.

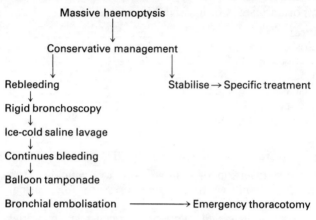

Figure 4.5 Scheme for management of massive haemoptysis

Infective exacerbations of chronic bronchitis

Chronic bronchitis is defined as cough, with sputum production on most days, for three consecutive months in 2 successive years. It is caused primarily by cigarette smoking.

The bronchial mucosa becomes oedematous and inflamed, mucous glands hypertrophy and secrete large quantities of tenacious mucus, and bronchial smooth muscle constricts. In addition, smoke denudes areas of cilia and inhibits ciliary motion so that sputum clearance is reduced.

Infective exacerbations are characterised by fever, increasing dyspnoea, wheeze and cough, producing increased volumes of purulent sputum. The commonest pathogens are *Haemophilus influenzae, Streptococcus pneumoniae* and *Branhamella catarrhalis*. Therefore, ampicillin (500 mg q.d.s.) is the drug of choice and, in cases of resistance, other alternatives are Augmentin (375 mg t.d.s.), co-trimoxazole or ciprofloxacin.

Eventually, poor alveolar ventilation gives rises to hypoxia and carbon dioxide retention, leading to pulmonary hypertension and right heart failure (cor pulmonale). The development of peripheral oedema in a patient with chronic bronchitis is an ominous prognostic sign. Most patients die within 5 years. These patients are 'blue and bloated'.

In health, there are two major drives to breathing: hypoxia and hypercarbia. When the lungs are no longer adequately ventilated, P_{CO_2} rises and hypercapnic drive is lost. The patient therefore breathes primarily because of the remaining hypoxic drive. If hypoxia is over-corrected with high inspired oxygen concentrations, the drive is lost. Clearly the oxygen concentration given must be carefully controlled by using an appropriate mask and it must be given continuously.

There are two types of mask:

1. *Ventimasks* employ a venturi device using the flow of oxygen to draw in a known amount of room air which is enriched and the enriched mixture then enters the mask. Thus 24, 28, 35 and 40% masks are available and the specified oxygen flow rate should be used with each mask.
2. *Edinburgh, Polymask, Hudson.* These general purpose masks rely on the patient's normal breathing pattern to draw in air to mix with the oxygen flowing into the enclosed space of the mask. If oxygen flow rate is increased, oxygen concentration rises. Clearly, if the patient has shallow respirations then not much air is drawn into the mask and the oxygen concentration automatically rises. These are excellent masks for postoperative patients but should never be used for controlled oxygen therapy as the patient's breathing is uncontrolled.

Oxygen may also be given through a nasal cannula. This form of oxygen delivery is most useful in patients requiring prolonged oxygen administration as it allows patients to talk and eat freely with oxygen flowing.

The actual concentration of inspired oxygen depends on the flow rate and the pattern of breathing, which determines how much mixing occurs in the nasopharynx. With normal breathing a flow of 2 litres per minute results in 24–28% concentration but when the patient is semi-stuporous the concentration can become dangerously high. Thus the ventimask is the only system which provides a guaranteed oxygen concentration.

Airflow obstruction may be improved with nebulised salbutamol (2.5–5.0 mg every two hours) and ipratropium bromide (2 ml every two hours). Most nebulisers require a high flow rate of oxygen to drive them. In CO_2-retaining patients this will abolish the hypoxic drive and they will stop breathing. Cylinders of compressed air must therefore be used to drive the nebulisers.

Apart from treatment of infection, inotropic support, diuretics and nebulised drugs, these patients need carefully planned oxygen therapy. The aim is a Po_2 of 7 kPa, as this puts the O_2 near the plateau on the oxygen dissociation curve without compromising hypoxic drive. Start with a 24% ventimask. Arterial blood gases should be checked after one hour. The Pco_2 may rise a little.

Providing the pH is not dropping (i.e. preferably > 7.25) and the patient is not becoming drowsy, simply observe events and repeat the blood gas after a further two hours. If tolerated, a 28% mask may be tried if the patient is still very hypoxic.

If he becomes drowsy on controlled oxygen and the Po_2 is less than 7 kPa, then an infusion of doxapram may be used. This acts as a respiratory stimulant and also improves V/Q mismatch in the lung. The usual range of dosage is 0.5–4.0 ml/min, assessing the gases every hour. Excess muscular activity, agitation and twitching indicate a need to reduce the dosage as this activity increases oxygen consumption. The dosage is further decreased after 12 hours providing infection has been controlled, a diuresis has been established and there is better air flow following nebulised bronchodilators. The infusion rate is lowered by 0.5 ml/min every 12 hours and aim to keep a Po_2 of 6.5–7.0 kPa or higher, and a pH of 7.25 or greater. Alkalosis, hypokalaemia or hypochloraemia due to diuretics should be sought and corrected.

Generally, chronic bronchitics do not respond to steroids. If the patient's history is not known, then i.v. hydrocortisone 100 mg q.d.s. or prednisolone 80 mg/day should be given in case there is an asthmatic component. Once the acute illness has resolved, all such patients should have a formal trial of steroids to assess responsiveness.

Ventilation

Patients with end-stage chronic bronchitis should not be ventilated. However, if the history is not known or the patient has a lobar pneumonia, ventilation may be considered.

The acute asthmatic attack

Asthma is defined as variable, reversible and generalised obstruction of airways, characterised by cough, dyspnoea and wheeze. An asthmatic attack may prove fatal. Underestimation of severity by patients and doctors, and the under-use of corticosteroids, may be responsible.

Three main mechanisms narrow the airways: bronchospasm, mucosal oedema and tenacious mucus plugging the main airways. 'All that wheezes is not asthma.' Foreign body, pulmonary oedema and pulmonary embolism must be excluded.

Severe asthma is indicated by:

- pulse rate higher than 110 beats per minute
- pulsus paradoxus higher than 20 mmHg
- PEFR less than 100 litres/min
- Normal or rising $P\text{CO}_2$.

An urgent chest X-ray excludes pneumonia or pneumothorax. Treat aggressively, closely monitoring progress, as follows:

- 60% humidified oxygen
- i.v. fluids to maintain intravascular volume and rehydrate
- potassium supplements
- if nebulisers are not available, give subcutaneously:
    adrenaline: 0.25–0.5 ml or 1:1000
    terbutaline: 0.25–0.5 mg 4-hourly
- if nebulisers are available:
    salbutamol: 2.5–5 mg 2-hourly
    ipratropium bromide: 0.5 mg 2–4-hourly
- hydrocortisone: 200 mg i.v. 6-hourly.
- prednisolone: 40 mg orally daily.

If the patient is still not improving, aminophylline is considered. The administration of this must be cautious, with a loading dose of 6 mg/kg over 30 min in infusion. Maintenance should be given according to Table 4.3. The theophylline level should be checked at 24 hours.

Table 4.3 Aminophylline maintenance dose (mg/kg/h)

	First 12 hours	Thereafter
Young smoker	1.18	0.94
Non-smoker	0.82	0.59
Cardiac failure and hepatic disease	0.71	0.35
Elderly and cor pulmonale	0.59	0.18

Most asthmatic attacks are precipitated by viral infection of the upper respiratory tract. Antibiotics should only be used if there is evidence of bacterial infection.

Close monitoring of patients is crucial. Ventilation is considered in cases of progressive confusion, exhaustion and rising $P\text{CO}_2$ and indicated in imminent death, with severe cyanosis, mental confusion, gasping, silent chest or cardiorespiratory arrest.

In extremely severe cases ether and halothane may be administered via the ventilator (as potent bronchodilators in refractory cases). Bronchial lavage is no longer recommended.

Inhalation of irritant gases

Many potentially dangerous gases or fumes are encountered in modern industry; their initial effects, when inhaled, are chemical inflammation of the terminal air passages and alveoli, and pulmonary oedema. Secondary infection may follow.

With very irritant gases the effects are immediate, resulting in watering of the eyes, sneezing, coughing and wheeze.

With phosgene (chlorine carbonyl) there is a latent period of up to 24 hours when pulmonary oedema occurs with no initial upper airways irritation. Patients must therefore be kept in for observation.

Exposure to hot smoke risks burns in the upper airways, manifesting as croup (laryngeal oedema) and wheeze. Smoke inhalation is common in house fires. Fibreoptic bronchoscopic inflammatory changes, consisting of oedema, sloughing or denuded mucosa, indicate direct thermal trauma rather than smoke injury, and these patients require early intubation. Thus, if a patient has facial burns the fibreoptic bronchoscope shows the severity of lower respiratory tract injury and may be used for the removal of retained secretions.

General principles of treatment

1. Remove to a safe area.
2. Remove contaminated clothing.
3. Ensure a clear airway.
4. Give:
   (a) high concentration humidified oxygen;
   (b) nebulised salbutamol 2.5 mg 2–4-hourly for wheeze;
   (c) i.v. hydrocortisone 200 mg q.i.d;
   (d) i.v. saline or plasma expanders if shocked;
   (e) antibiotics to cover any infection.
5. ? Bronchoscope in smoke inhalation.
6. May need to intubate and give positive pressure ventilation.

In the long term, after an acute injury, the lungs may go on to develop obliterative bronchiolitis or heal with interstitial pulmonary fibrosis.

The lungs in systemic disease

The following multisystem diseases may affect the lungs to a greater or lesser degree. Autoimmune screen, antinuclear factor and rhesus factor should always be checked in collagen diseases.

Rheumatoid arthritis

1. Pleural effusion or pericardial effusion – exudate with low glucose level.
2. Rheumatoid nodules similar to those found on elbows may be seen on chest X-ray and may be mistaken for metastatic carcinoma. May cavitate.
3. Interstitial pulmonary fibrosis – may respond to high-dose steroids.

Systemic lupus erythematosus

1. Pleurisy and pericarditis.
2. Interstitial pulmonary fibrosis.
3. Pulmonary embolism.

Scleroderma

1. The most likely to give interstitial fibrosis.
2. Oesophageal dysmotility may lead to recurrent aspiration pneumonia.

Sarcoidosis

This typically presents with bilateral hilar lymphadenopathy; a large majority recover without therapy. Patients may progress to interstitial pulmonary fibrosis. Other systems to remember are: parotids, eyes, brain, pituitary, heart, joints, skin, e.g. lupus pernio, erythema nodosum, bone cysts.

Systemic steroids are mandatory for treating ocular, CNS and pituitary complications and hypercalcaemia.

Diagnosis is established by a positive Kveim test (0.15 Kveim reagent intradermal; biopsy at 6 weeks: granulomas in the biopsy are diagnostic. Not positive in 50–60%); or at fibreoptic bronchoscopy when granulomas are found in the bronchial mucosa or transbronchial lung biopsy; or by biopsy of skin lesion; or by biopsy of lymph nodes.

Serum angiotensin converting enzyme may be of value in monitoring clinical activity.

Important differential diagnosis: tuberculosis; Hodgkin's disease.

Wegener's granulomatosis

The triad of upper airways disease, e.g. sinusitis, mucosal ulceration, perforated nasal septum, renal casts or red cells, and pulmonary nodules.

The diagnosis may be made by renal biopsy or biopsy of the pulmonary nodules. Serum neutrophil cytoplasmic antibody may prove to be a useful test for monitoring disease progress (send 10 ml clotted blood to immunology).

Treatment

Cyclophosphamide 100 mg/day orally; prednisolone 20 mg/day orally.

Other systems involved:

- joints (56%)
- skin/muscle (44%)
- eyes (39%)
- middle ear (39%)
- heart (28%)
- CNS (22%).

Polyarteritis nodosa

This can present as asthma with eosinophilia. At one end of the spectrum is the Churg–Strauss syndrome which involves skin lesions (vasculitic), peripheral nerves, myocardium, pulmonary infiltrates; renal failure is less common than with PN.

Tests

- ESR (high)
- WBC count (eosinophilia)
- microscopy of urine
- renal biopsy or skin biopsy
- coeliac angiograms.

Treatment

Prednisolone 40–60 mg/day; azathioprin 50 mg t.d.s. or cyclophosphamide.

Goodpasture's syndrome

A syndrome combining pulmonary haemorrhage and glomer-ulonephritis. Immune complexes are deposited on basement membrane of the kidney and lung. Immunofluorescent staining for IgG gives a characteristic pattern.

Treatment
Plasma exchange plus immunosuppressive drugs.

The natural history of the disease is gradual loss of circulating antibodies over 6 months to several years; this may be accelerated by treatment.

Cystic fibrosis

This is the commonest fatal inherited (recessive) disease; it affects about 6000 patients in the UK. It used to be a paediatric disease but with improved therapy 80% are expected to reach their 16th birthday.

Diagnosis is confirmed by a sweat test. Sodium concentration in sweat over 60 mmol/litre in children or 80 mmol/litre on two occasions in adults is diagnostic.

Main problems

Lungs

1. Recurrent infection with *Staph. aureus* or *Pseudomonas aeruginosa*.
2. Eventually respiratory failure – consider lung transplant.

Always culture sputum. Treatment:

1. Flucloxacillin 2–3 g q.d.s. for *Staph. aureus*.
2. Azlocillin plus gentamicin or ceftazidime or ciprofloxacin for pseudomonas.
3. Pneumothorax – common – usual treatment.
4. Massive haemoptysis (10%) – majority settle with conservative management; – if recurrent, bronchial arterial embolisation performed. May need to resect lobe.

Pancreas
Malabsorption, especially of fat, leads to malnutrition. Treatment: pancreatic enzyme supplements (Creon) 2–3 capsules with each meal. Coating dissolves in less acid environment of small bowel releasing the enzymes. Add H_2 blocker to decrease acidity if

steatorrhoea persists. Twenty per cent become diabetic; treat with insulin.

Other important complications

- male infertility 100%
- sinusitis 90%
- nasal polyps 10–20%
- diabetes 10–20%
- distal intestinal obstruction 10–20%
- gall stones 10%
- portal hypertension 10%
- aspergillosis 10%.

Principles of treatment

- appropriate large doses of antibiotics
- physiotherapy
- physical exercise a valuable adjunct
- diet and nutrition – at least 150% of recommended diet for a normal person; enteric coated microspheres of pancreatic enzymes; H_2 blocker to decrease acidity if steatorrhoea persists.
- psychological counselling
- ?lung transplantation.

Pneumonia

There has been a change in the pattern of infecting organisms seen both in the community and in hospital practice since the advent of the antibiotic era. In association with this, the development of a very large spectrum of antibiotics has enabled treatment of pneumonias which in the past have been associated with a very high mortality.

Classification

The lobar and bronchopneumonia of the old classification tends to merge with many modern-day infections. Lobar consolidation may rapidly develop into diffuse bronchopneumonia. Classification may predict the causative organism and therefore indicate treatment early. An arbitrary classification allows a 'best guess' at aetiology but this should not be taken as a rigid guide. Isolation of the organisms is necessary for correct treatment.

Community acquired

1. *Primary bacterial.* The principal bacterial infection remains the pneumococcus, particularly if the patient presents with lobar pneumonia.
2. *Associated with chronic obstructive airways disease.* Principal infecting oranisms: klebsiella, viral and *Haemophilus influenzae.*
3. *Viral.* Common in children and patients with pre-existing pulmonary disease. May also be seen in patients, previously fit, during outbreaks with virulent strains, particularly influenza virus.
4. *Primary atypical.* The principal organisms are mycoplasma and legionella. The latter usually occurs in outbreaks but may occur in isolated cases.

Hospital acquired

1. *Aspiration pneumonia.* Usually associated with depressed conscious level and depressed reflexes but may not be associated with obvious vomiting. Organisms are variable but virtually always include anaerobic Gram-negative bacilli.
2. *'Hypostatic'.* Following debilitating illnesses, or as a result of sputum retention, e.g. in neuromuscular diseases with poor cough, and postabdominal surgery as a result of diaphragmatic splinting from pain or abdominal distension. Organisms vary according to the clinical circumstance and no single organism predominates.
3. *Secondary acquired infection (nosocomial).* This is commonly seen in intensive care units and incidences rise rapidly with duration of stay in the unit. Over one week, virtually all patients develop secondary infection. The main organisms responsible are aerobic Gram-negative bacilli and fungi or candida.

Opportunistic

Found in immunocompromised patients whatever the aetiology. This subject is dealt with separately (see p. 247).

Clinical presentations

1. *Dyspnoea.* Usually the first clinical sign but usually associated with significant biochemical and radiological changes.

2. *Increasing hypoxia.* The course of these diseases is very variable from a slowly progressive hypoxia to a fulminant course requiring intervention, occasionally within hours of presentation.
3. *Sputum production.* Also very variable depending on the underlying agent. Examination of the sputum is essential and every effort should be made to obtain samples. The ability to expectorate often determines the point of intervention.
4. *X-ray.* The radiological findings reflect the extent of the disease but severe pneumonia, whatever the aetiology, may result in identical radiological consolidation.
5. *Bacteriology.* A direct Gram smear of sputum will confirm the presence of bacteria and the clinical circumstances will indicate the likely causative organism but definitive diagnosis can only be obtained on culture of sputum. It may be necessary to resort to transtracheal aspiration to obtain samples or to attempt sputum induction via various inhalations. The diversity of organisms that may produce pneumonia, particularly in hospital practice, makes co-operation with a microbiologist essential.

Treatment

Specific therapy consists of antibiotics, as determined from sputum culture and sensitivity findings from isolated organisms. 'Best guess' treatment is determined by the clinical circumstances in which the pneumonia arises and should be reviewed regularly, according to sputum isolates.

Clinical assessment

Between 8 and 20% of patients from various studies presenting with community acquired pneumonia still die. Factors indicting severe pneumonia which should actively be sought are:

- hypoxia
- respiratory rate higher than 30/min
- leukocytosis
- leukopenia
- diastolic pressure lower than 60 mmHg
- raised urea
- hypoalbuminaemia
- arrhythmias (atrial fibrillation).

Respiratory failure is the indication for ventilation.

Lung abscess

This is a necrotic, often encapsulated and cavitated mass of infected lung tissue. Important causes are:

1. Aspiration (general anaesthesia, alcoholism, central nervous system injuries and general debilitation). The main micro-organisms are anaerobic: *Bacteroides fragilis, Fusobacterium nucleatum,* etc.
2. Postpneumonic (alcoholics, immunosuppressed, diabetics, cancer patients, renal failure and transplantation). Micro-organisms are *Klebsiella pneumoniae,* pseudomonas, *Staphylococcus aureus* and streptococcus. Sometimes there is no specific cause.
3. Secondary to regional or distant sepsis (carcinoma, sequestration, broncho-oesophageal fistulae, foreign bodies, pulmonary infarction).

The clinical presentation is often with foul sputum, radiologically localised opacities, cavitation, necrotising pneumonia and pyopneumothorax. Bacteriology is obtained from sputum, transtracheal or percutaneous needle aspiration.

Management is based on antibiotics, evacuation of pus, and drainage; resection of necrotic tissues only if necessary. First-line antibiotics are penicillin G, metronidazole and cephalosporins. Thereafter, according to bacteriological advice.

Drainage can be performed by bronchoscopy, or externally when the lung is thoroughly adherent to the pleura. A tube suffices if the pus is thin, but very thick pus necessitates open drainage. Pulmonary resection is required if there is associated malignancy.

Secondary complications such as empyema or bronchopleural fistula are treated on their merits.

Pulmonary infection in the immunocompromised patient

In immunodepressed patients, cough, dyspnoea, fever and a pulmonary infiltrate on chest X-rays could mean: extension of primary disease, drug reaction, pulmonary haemorrhage, common bacterial infection, fungi, parasites or viruses.

In every episode of suspected pulmonary infection a complete set of tests must be done: full blood count, platelets, prothrombin-time, viral titres, blood cultures, sputum for Gram stain and cultures. More invasive tests in particular cases are: fibreoptic bronchoscopy, transtracheal aspiration, and lung biopsy (percutaneous or open).

Some clues present on chest X-rays help the diagnosis: localised opacities associated with cavitation may indicate bacterial infection, septic emboli and aspergillus; lobar consolidation plus cavity indicate Gram-negative or anaerobic infection; miliary infiltrate can be caused by rapidly progressive tuberculosis; bilateral diffuse infiltrates may indicate *Pneumocystis carinii,* cytomegalovirus or drug reaction. If a bacterial infection is suspected, broad spectrum cover should be given whilst awaiting culture. Two regimes are: ceftazidime + metronidazole; ampicillin + gentamicin + metronidazole. If legionella is a possibility: erythromycin + rifampicin.

Extension of the primary disease is present in Hodgkin's disease, lymphosarcoma and systemic lupus erythematosus.

Drug reaction may be due to busulphan, cyclophosphamide, melphalan, bleomycin and methotrexate.

It must be noted that several pathogens may coexist.

Opportunistic pulmonary infections

History

The recognition of opportunistic lung infections is a relatively recent phenomenon. The development of powerful anticancer drugs, the recognition of and ability to treat various diseases associated with the immunocompromised state, and the tremendous increase in organ transplantation and its associated control of the immune system has allowed previously non-pathogenic organisms to produce significant disease. In recent times, the prevalence of the acquired immune deficiency syndrome (AIDS) has *increased* the frequency of pulmonary infection with organisms hitherto thought unimportant.

Clinical features

1. *Severe progressive hypoxia.* A slight initial fall in arterial Po_2 may progress, at variable speed, to significant hypoxia on 100% oxygen and the rate of deterioration is not related to the causative organism. It is not unknown for patients to go from normal oxygenation to death from hypoxia within 2–3 days. Hypercapnia (type II respiratory failure) is a relatively late phenomenon.
2. *Dyspnoea.* Mild dyspnoea is usually the first clinical symptom, following a significant fall in Po_2. This finding may also precede other clinical features.

3. *Clinical examination.* Apart from occasional diffuse crepitations, examination is non-contributory.
4. *Sputum.* This is usually produced in very small amounts, if any, and on appearance is non-purulent. Haemoptysis is uncommon.
5. *Chest X-ray.* This will show diffuse pulmonary opacities in both lung fields, indistinguishable from those seen in acute pulmonary oedema, ARDS, etc. The most striking aspect of the X-ray is that the severity of changes seem disproportionate to the amount of functional deterioration.
6. *Systemic effects.* Opportunistic infection is usually associated with minimal systemic disturbances. In particular, pyrexia is uncommon and patients do not appear toxic. This is presumably because the patient is unable to mount a significant inflammatory response.
7. The clinical circumstances of immune suppression or organ transplantation.

Causative organisms

Any organism may produce the same clinical picture. The most commonly encountered organisms are:

1. Bacteria: Gram-negative rods, Gram-positive cocci, legionella.
2. Viruses: cytomegalovirus, herpes, varicella zoster.
3. Protozoa: pneumocystis, toxoplasma.
4. Others: aspergillus, candida.

The pattern of infecting organisms has changed with changing immunosuppression following organ transplantation. Pre-cyclosporin, the most common infecting organisms after cardiac transplantation were pneumocystis, aspergillus, CMV and the herpes viruses. With the advent of cyclosporin, there has been a significant fall in the incidence of the first three but a significant increase in infections with legionella in particular.

Investigations

'Blanket' antibiotic therapy against all possible organisms is impossible, so accurate identification of the infective agent is indispensable.

1. *Examination of sputum.* This rarely will give a diagnosis in this situation. Bacteria isolated may be secondary infections and the amount of sputum produced is usually very small.

2. *Induction of sputum.* This has been attempted using inhalation of steam or other agents and samples obtained by either expectoration or transtracheal aspiration. A high return in terms of isolation of pneumocystis has been found in patients with AIDS but its value is limited in other infections.
3. *Bronchoscopy* with bronchial washings or brushings. This has the disadvantage of requiring an invasive procedure, often with sedation, in someone who is hypoxic. In the early stage of the disease, under proper clinical and anaesthetic control, it is safe and can give the diagnosis. There is a recognised morbidity, and resuscitation and intubation equipment must be available.
4. *Lung biopsy.* This may be carried out via the bronchoscope or open, through a small thoracotomy. Both procedures are associated with a significant but small morbidity, in particular pulmonary haemorrhage and pneumothorax. Open lung biopsy gives an adequate specimen of lung under direct vision, is very well tolerated and has the highest chance of a positive diagnosis.

Respiratory emergencies in cancer

Lung cancer kills about 30 000 people a year in the UK and its care forms a large proportion of the chest physician's and surgeon's work. Only 25% of patients are operable after fairly simple assessment and only nine or ten cases out of a hundred are 'curable' by surgery. However, 80% of small-cell cancers will have a response and improved survival with chemotherapy. Median survival from diagnosis of untreated small-cell cancer is 6 weeks, but with present chemotherapy regimes a median survival of 11 months can be hoped for, with some longer survivors. Chemotherapy has not been successful for non-small-cell lung cancer.

The respiratory emergencies in cancer may be disease related or therapy related.

Disease-related emergencies

1. *SVC obstruction.* Remember not all SVC obstruction is due to lung cancer; lymphoma or aneurysm amongst others can also produce this. However, histological diagnosis may have to wait. The patient has a suffused face with distended non-pulsatile neck veins and perhaps oedematous arms. High-dose prednisolone 40 mg/day and radiotherapy are first line strategems. However, if the patient is known to have small-cell lung cancer then chemotherapy can relieve obstruction as quickly.

2. *Massive haemoptysis.* This dramatic emergency may need rigid bronchoscopy to see the site of bleeding. Local adrenaline may be more appropriate if the bleed is torrential. For lesser bleeds radiotherapy is effective, transfusion may be required.

3. *Central airway occlusion.* This may be difficult to diagnose as a small, critically-placed tracheal tumour may not be visible on chest X-ray. Bronchoscopy is required on suspicion of such a tumour. However, biopsy may have to be deferred if the tracheal lumen is threatened. Radiotherapy may help as may chemotherapy in small-cell carcinoma (remember sputum cytology may be obtained if you cannot biopsy). Where available, laser therapy to a central lesion is very effective. Symptomatic relief may be obtained by giving the patient a helium–oxygen mixture and high-dose corticosteroid. Flow/volume loops can help distinguish intrathoracic from extrathoracic central occlusion (see lung function tests). With an extrathoracic occlusion tracheostomy may be life-sparing.

4. *Pulmonary embolus.* This life-threatening disorder can be very difficult to diagnose and its presence should always be considered. If the patient is terminal, symptomatic treatment with oxygen and opiates is required. Pulmonary emboli may need streptokinase via pulmonary arterial catheters. Small emboli can pass unnoticed and lead to steady, unexplained deterioration. Lung scans may be difficult to interpret postoperatively or in the presence of tumour, but multiple defects of perfusion unmatched on ventilation scan help the diagnosis.

5. *Massive pleural effusion.* This may be due to bleeding or metastases. If this is leading to mediastinal shift, insert a large drain and drain off a little fluid and clamp (over-rapid drainage and re-expansion of collapsed lung may lead to unilateral pulmonary oedema). On draining to dryness, installation of tetracyclines or corynebacterium may prevent recurrence.

6. *Lymphatic carcinomatosis.* This leads to progressive and acute breathlessness as tumour invades along pulmonary vessels and lymphatics, giving bilateral bullous enlargement with streaky shadows fanning out into the lungs. This is more associated with mammary and gastric carcinomas than pulmonary tumour. Therapy is symptomatic with oxygen and opiates.

7. *Cardiac tamponade.* May occur with cardiac invasion or pericardial effusion and may require pericardial drainage.

With all these emergencies the overall prognosis of the patient has to be taken into account and a balance has to be found between nihilism and rigid following of protocol.

Therapy-related problems

1. *Postoperative emergencies.*
2. *Chemotherapy* can render the patient particularly susceptible to infection which may be atypical in immunosupressed patients. First think of conventional chest infection due to pneumococcus and *Haemophilus influenzae*. Rarer problems may be as in other immunosupressed patients (see p. 247). Chemotherapy can lead to infiltration of the lung itself, so it is important to have precise details of chemotherapy regimens. Bleomycin can cause pulmonary fibrosis which is irreversible.
3. *Radiotherapy* may cause a pneumonitis, although shielding of the normal lung is practised. This is dose related and field specific so details of the radiotherapy should be sought. Pneumonitis takes months to develop and treatment is symptomatic. The distinction from recurrence of tumour can be difficult.

The most important aspect of the management of the cancer patient is communication. Patients are probably more frightened of the manner than of the fact of death. Anticipate the questions and assure the patient that he should not have pain (this is true!). Remember above all that not all respiratory problems in patients with lung cancer are due to the tumour. Such patients (generally being smokers) get myocardial infarctions, pulmonary emboli and perforated ulcers and are too often assumed to be 'terminal'.

Nursing aspects of thoracic procedures

Tracheostomy

Every effort is made to avoid infection of a sternotomy wound from a tracheostomy, which is delayed wherever possible until the mediastinum is better 'sealed'. The procedure is explained to the patient if he is able to understand. The relatives must also be informed and consent for operation obtained. Blood should be cross-matched.

A chest X-ray will be taken soon after the patient returns to intensive care. The tracheostomy tube will be suctioned as necessary and the type and amount of tracheal aspirate recorded. At first the secretions may be fairly heavily blood stained, but should become less blood stained within a few hours of returning to ITU.

The size of the tracheostomy is noted in the nursing care plan and a tube of the same make and size and a pair of tracheal dilators kept at the bedside in case of emergency. The tracheostomy dressing is changed as often as necessary. This may be several times in 24 hours. Each time the tube is cleared by suction the area around the tracheostomy is also cleaned. The stoma is cleaned with Chlorasol and dried. A dry dressing is applied. The tapes holding the tracheostomy tube in place should be kept clean and secure.

The tracheostomy tube will be renewed at least every 7 days by the surgeon.

Mini-tracheostomy

Requirements

- mini-tracheostomy pack containing tube, blades, suction catheter
- dressing pack and anaesthetic
- local anaesthetic with syringe and needle
- suction apparatus
- size 8 suction catheters
- theatre light.

Procedure

1. Reassure the patient.
2. Position patient: upright with a pillow under shoulders with head back and neck extended. Make sure that the patient is comfortable as it is important that he remains in this position until the procedure is completed.
3. Check suction apparatus is working and connect suction catheter.
4. Ensure there is a good light-source.
5. Assist surgeon carrying out the procedure.
6. Once mini-tracheostomy is *in situ,* secure it with tapes.
7. 'Suction' tube: record amount and type of secretions.
8. Spigot mini-tracheostomy tube and give oxygen as required via face mask.
9. Make patient comfortable at the end of procedure.
10. Send sputum daily for culture and sensitivity.

Bronchoscopy

This procedure may be quite distressing if not properly explained to the patient, particularly fibreoptic bronchoscopy under local anaesthesia. A complete set for cardiac arrest must be kept to hand.

Requirements

- bronchoscopy tray
- light-source
- intubation equipment
- insufflator
- sterile water
- KY jelly
- sputum specimen trap
- suction apparatus
- sedation, as prescribed by the doctor.

Procedure

1. Explain to the patient.
2. Sedate.
3. Attach insufflator to oxygen supply.
4. Connect light-source to correct bronchoscope.
5. Lubricate bronchoscope.
6. Connect suction catheter and specimen trap to suction apparatus.
7. Use sterile water to flush suction equipment.
8. Lie patient flat with pillow under shoulders and neck extended.
9. Observe patient's heart rate and blood pressure.
10. Send sputum for culture and sensitivity.
11. Order chest X-rays.
12. Make patient comfortable following procedure.

Thoracic surgery

Cardiothoracic trauma

Trauma is the third most common cause of death in the Western world, exceeded only by cancer and cardiovascular disease. In the USA it is the leading cause of death in people below the age of 45. Cardiothoracic trauma causes a quarter of all of the avoidable deaths.

Mechanism of injury

Chest trauma can be caused by blunt, penetrating, blast or thermal mechanisms.

Penetrating chest injury

In bullet injury, damage occurs owing to the transfer of kinetic energy from the missile to the chest. The energy is usually transferred over a small volume of tissue. Kinetic energy (KE) is determined by the formula:

$$KE = \frac{1}{2}mv^2$$

where m = mass of the missile, and v is the velocity of the missile.

It can be seen that the velocity of impact is the most important factor in determining the degree of tissue damage. Low-velocity missiles, such as knives, cause laceration and crushing of tissues in their path. High-velocity missiles (classified as travelling at speeds of higher than 500 m/s) cause similar damage but also exhibit cavitation and shock-wave formation as they travel through the tissue, creating widespread destruction, depending on the tissue density and elasticity. Ballistic missiles rarely travel in a straight line within the body as they are deflected by bone and fascial planes. The course of the missile and extent of tissue damage cannot therefore be predicted simply from knowledge of the site of entry and angle of penetration.

High-velocity missile injuries create cavitation in their path. Clothing, skin and destroyed tissue are sucked into the path of the missile, causing gross contamination.

The following injuries may result from the penetrating trauma:

- pneumothorax
- haemothorax
- pulmonary laceration
- pulmonary haematoma
- penetrating vascular injury
- penetrating cardiac injury
- penetrating oesophageal injury.

Blunt chest injury

Kinetic energy is distributed over a larger area than in penetrating trauma. There is direct deformation of tissue at the site of impact. Rapid acceleration or deceleration of the chest results in compression, stretching and shearing of tissues at points of anatomical fixation. These forces cause damage in relation to their kinetic energy. The intima of the aorta within the chest is particularly susceptible to shearing forces and will tear at the isthmus at the site of its fixation.

The following injuries may result from blunt trauma:

- puncture by rib
- sternal fracture
- flail chest
- pneumothorax
- haemothorax
- tracheobronchial disruption
- pulmonary contusion
- aortic rupture
- myocardial contusions
- cardiac rupture
- ruptured valve
- septal defects
- diaphragmatic rupture.

Blast injury to the lung

There are four mechanisms involved in 'blast lung'.

1. High pressure shock wave following the explosions. The magnitude of tissue damage due to this decreases rapidly as the distance from the explosion increases.

2. Negative pressure wave. This follows the high pressure wave and is of a lower amplitude.

These two pressure waves cause compression and expansion of the lung parenchyma.

3. Shearing forces, secondary to non-uniform application of (1) and (2) throughout the chest.
4. Bubble formation at the air–fluid interface of the pulmonary parenchyma as the pressure waves flow across the alveolar–capillary membranes.

Thermal injury

The following mechanisms are involved:

1. The patient may suffer anoxia due to low oxygen concentration in vicinity of fires.
2. Oedema and obstruction of the upper airway secondary to the heat.
3. Free-radical release within the pulmonary microcirculation secondary to hypoxia. Subsequently the damaged capillary membranes leak high-protein-content fluid into the intersitium.
4. Inhalation of noxious gases released by the fire.
5. Bronchospasm secondary to (1)–(4).
6. Thoracic eschar formations restricting ventilation.

General pulmonary damage in severe trauma

It is well recognised that in severe cases of trauma there is always some amount of pulmonary impairment. This results from a variety of factors which all eventually cause a leak of red blood cells and high-protein-containing fluid into the pulmonary interstitium and eventually the aleveoli. In its gross form this is recognised as shock lung or adult respiratory distress syndrome. It is, however, probable that there is some damage to the pulmonary capillary membrane in all forms of trauma.

The aetiological factors are:

• inadequate analgesia causing splinting and atelectasis
• pneumonia
• pulmonary emboli
• inhalation of vomit/noxious fumes
• overzealous transfusion
• fat emboli
• oxygen toxicity

- transfusion reactions
- generalised sepsis.

One or more of these factors may lead to capillary membrane damage.

Effect of injury

Chest injuries may be classified as:

1. Rapidly fatal: implies instantaneous death or death within minutes and accounts for 50% of fatalities from thoracic trauma.
2. Potentially lethal: accounts for remaining 50% of deaths; 30% within hours of injury (usually because of haemorrhage), 20% days or weeks later (from sepsis or multi-system organ failure).
3. Not fatal.

Little can be done to reduce fatalities in the first group apart from legislative preventative measures. Much can be done, however, to reduce death in the second group using rapid transfer to hospital and improved management.

Emergency management of the patient with a chest injury

1. Initial evaluation.
2. Subsequent early management.
3. Emergency surgery.

Initial evaluation

The airway is cleared and maintained. If ventilation appears inadequate the patient is intubated and ventilated.

Open pneumothorax, tension pneumothorax, flail chest or pericardial tamponade should be looked for. If present they require instant management (see below).

A rapid examination is made of the patient: pulse, blood pressure, skin perfusion, brief auscultation of both sides of the chest, neck veins, abdomen, search for major external haemorrhage, and rapid neurological assessment (pupils, eye opening, verbal response, motor response).

Blood is taken for cross-matching through a large-bore i.v. cannula. If the patient is hypotensive, a rapid infusion of crystalloid is begun. This is stopped when the pressure returns to greater than 100 mmHg systolic or when 2 litres have been infused and thus the need for further volume reassessed.

External haemorrhage is controlled using direct pressure. Fractures are splinted.

Subsequent early management

A history is obtained from any witness available.

Blood is taken for blood gas estimation, packed cell volume, and acid–base evaluation.

A complete and detailed examination of the patient is made, including the back. At all times the possibility of a cervical injury should be borne in mind and extension/flexion avoided, if appropriate, with a collar.

Persisting hypotension (<100 mmHg systolic) is an indication for CVP line insertion, urinary catheterisation and blood transfusion, if necessary using unmatched, type-specific blood.

A chest X-ray is an essential requirement. It should always be performed prior to insertion of an intercostal drain unless tension pneumothorax is suspected. The physical signs are respiratory distress, mediastinal shift and diminished breath sounds on the affected side, associated with hypotension. It is treated by immediate insertion of a wide-bore cannula in the second intercostal space anteriorly. If the diagnosis is correct there will be a rush of air accompanied by relief of symptoms. A chest X-ray is then obtained prior to lateral insertion of an intercostal drain.

Patients with blunt trauma should have a 12-lead ECG and all patients should be connected to an ECG monitor.

Emergency surgery

The following patients should have instant thoracotomy in the emergency room of casualty:

1. Patients in cardiac arrest following chest trauma.
2. Patients with persisting and deteriorating hypotension, despite volume administration and adequate control of the airway and ventilation, following penetrating chest trauma.
3. Patients with evidence of cardiac tamponade following blunt or penetrating trauma. The signs are:
   (a) hypokinesis;
   (b) distended neck veins with elevated JVP;
   (c) central trachea;
   (d) ± penetrating chest wound, typically over the precordium.

The following are required to perform an emergency thoracotomy:

1. Courage.
2. A scalpel.
3. Skin-prep to be poured over the chest immediately prior to incision.
4. An anaesthetist.
5. At least one good swab with a sterile end.
6. Any member of staff as an assistant.

The following are not absolutely necessary, but make the task much easier. They are all that it is necessary to include in an emergency thoracotomy set in casualty. Such a set should be made up by the staff from cardiothoracic theatres and changed at least at monthly intervals:

- 1 rib spreader
- 1 pair dissecting scissors
- 1 needle holder
- 1 soft vascular clamp
- 2 large Roberts forceps
- 4/0 Prolene suture
- size 30 Foley catheter
- surgical drapes
- internal defibrillator paddles.

A good light source and previous experience make an enormous difference.

The patient is rolled slightly to the right. The skin, underlying muscle and intercostal muscles are incised in the line of the fourth intercostal space from the anterior axillary line to the sternal edge, and then spread using the hands and subsequently the chest spreader if available. Pericardial tamponade will be apparent by a disturbed, discoloured, haemorrhagic pericardium. To the inexperienced this looks like the ventricle, but must be the pericardium. When incised, clot will be encountered. The pericardium should be cut in the line of the phrenic nerve, anterior to it, from apex to pulmonary artery. The pressure may rise, the CVP will fall. Penetrating injury of the heart can be controlled with light digital pressure.

The patient is then transferred to theatre.

Management of specific chest injuries

Rapidly lethal lesions

Airway obstruction
Note patency of nose and mouth, intercostal retraction, quality of respiratory movements and obvious signs of respiratory distress.

Extract foreign bodies from the mouth and lift the jaws, provided that there is no cervical fracture, to keep the airway free from obstruction. If the patient is unconscious, an oral airway should be inserted. If there is respiratory insufficiency, intubate.

Tension pneumothorax

Pulmonary collapse, shifting of the mediastinum to the contra-lateral side, lowering of venous return and severe haemodynamic compromise are all indications of this condition. Clinically, respiratory distress, lack of ventilatory movements, cyanosis, distant cardiac sounds and bulky hemithorax indicate increased intrathoracic tension. Treatment is the immediate drainage of air.

Open pneumothorax

Pendeluft produces increased effective dead space. Limited ventilatory capacity, lowered venous return and mediastinal movement cause haemodynamic deterioration.

Massive haemothorax

More than 2000 ml of blood in the pleural cavity. Mortality rate is 4% when it is associated with penetrating trauma and nearly 50% when the cause is blunt trauma. It usually presents with hypovolaemic shock, severe hypoventilation and clinical signs of pleural effusion. One litre of blood is the minimum perceptible in supine chest X-rays. Treatment includes fluid infusion, blood transfusion, thoracic drainage and thoracotomy when indicated. The indications for surgery are: deep shock; more than 2000 ml of blood collected within the first 4 hours after trauma; more than 200 ml of blood through the thoracic drain every hour for 4 consecutive hours; and more than 400 ml of blood in any hour.

Flail chest

A segment of chest wall in anatomical and functional discontinuity with the rest of the thoracic cage, because of multiple fractures, restricts pulmonary parenchyma, increases ventilatory work and dead space, and dimishes tidal volume and oxygen transport. The initial treatment is pressure to stop paradoxical movement. Oxygen and aggressive analgesia may obviate ventilatory support. Mechanical ventilation may become necessary if there is need of general anaesthesia for other reasons; associated pulmonary contusion, trauma of the central nervous system and signs of progressive respiratory failure. Where prolonged ventilation is poorly supervised, surgical fixation of the flail segment may enable the patient to be nursed successfully in normal wards.

Cardiac tamponade

In blunt trauma is generally lethal. In penetrating trauma a cardiac wound must be suspected in any epigastric or parasternal wound. The clinical picture includes distant heart sounds, high venous pressure and hypotension. In some cases the patient is in deep shock and a paradoxical pulse can be detected. In some doubtful cases, if the patient is stable enough, fluoroscopy or echocardiography demonstrate the intrapericardial fluid. Sometimes pericardiocentesis can be used as a temporary measure to avoid severe haemodynamic compromise in the emergency room until the patient has a definitive operation.

Potentially lethal lesions

Pulmonary contusion

Mainly related to blunt trauma when the glottis is closed. The seriousness varies from the small lung haematoma to the so-called 'traumatic lung' that usually appears after the initial trauma. What really impairs the prognosis in these patients is fluid overloading. Therefore intravenous fluids should be limited up to 1000 ml in the initial resuscitation and to 30 ml/kg/day the next 72 hours (provided there is not any associated lesion requiring different treatment). Also frusemide, analgesia, physiotherapy and methylprednisolone are part of the management.

Aortic rupture

Just 15% of these patients reach the hospital. Sub-total rupture at the left subclavian artery level is the commonest situation. A high-speed blunt injury in a young patient, with chest X-ray with signs of widening of the upper mediastinum, possible deviation of the left main bronchus and tracheal bifurcation, supraclavicular opacity, or obliteration of the normal cardiac contour, should indicate an aortogram and prompt surgical repair or replacement of the damaged segment, usually the isthmus of the aorta.

Tracheobronchial rupture

Results from tracheal compression against the spine, distension of the airways with closed glottis and hypertension of the bronchial tree. Fractures of the larynx produce dysphonia and subcutaneous emphysema. The majority of lesions of the bronchi occur at 2.5 cm from the carina, and the clinical picture depends on the degree of communication between the ruptured segment and the pleural space; pneumothorax refractory to conventional treatment, pneumomediastinum, haemoptysis and signs of respiratory failure can be present. There may be linear tears or complete transection and crushing. Bronchoscopic diagnosis should be followed by surgical repair. Cardiopulmonary bypass may be helpful when both main bronchi are transected.

Oesophageal rupture
Epigastric trauma may rupture the lower third of the oesophagus; vomiting of an overfilled stomach against a closed glottis may split the oesophagus from top to bottom (Boerhaave). In both situations there is upper abdominal pain, cervical emphysema, dysphagia and sometimes gastrointestinal bleeding and early sepsis due to mediastinitis. A contrast swallow with hydrosoluble medium and in some cases oesophagoscopy confirm the diagnosis. The treatment is surgical and, depending on the time elapsed, primary suture, oesophageal exclusion or oesophageal resection may be performed.

Diaphragmatic rupture
More frequent on the left side. The clinical picture may range from total absence of symptoms to different degrees of shock. There is abdominal pain, hypotension and chest X-rays showing diaphragmatic elevation, gas of an abnormal pattern within the chest and displacement of a nasogastric tube. The spleen may be visible above the diaphragm. Treatment is surgical.

Myocardial contusion
This occurs in at least 20% of severe thoracic trauma. The surgical pathology and the clinical picture is that of myocardial ischaemia, as is the treatment: close monitoring and arrhythmia control, as well as improvement of low cardiac output.

Lesions not immediately life threatening

These include well-tolerated degrees of haemothorax, pneumothorax, soft-tissue injuries, intrathoracic foreign bodies and bone fractures. So-called 'single-rib fractures' can be very dangerous if overlooked. They are frequently associated with pulmonary contusion and the pain may impair ventilatory mechanics. The mortality rate in single-rib fractures in patients over 80 years is about 20%. Patients at risk are: elderly, chronic respiratory patients, and those with associated pleural effusion. Treatment is local anaesthetic with lignocaine 1%. Injuries to the first and second ribs, as well as scapular and sternal fractures, might be associated with severe intrathoracic injuries.

Empyema thoracis

Empyema is the accumulation of pus in a natural cavity. In the pleura it usually has three phases:

1. Exudative, with thin fluid, low cellular content and frequently negative culture.
2. Fibrinopurulent, with fibrin, polymorphonuclear cells and more viscous fluid.
3. Organising, with thick fluid, pus and fibroblasts.

Later still, the empyema may point through the chest wall as 'empyema necessitans' and there may be loculation trapping the lung.

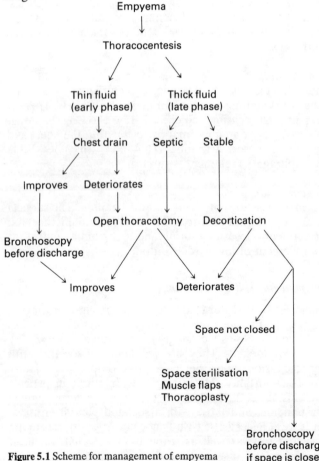

Figure 5.1 Scheme for management of empyema

The aetiology can be:

1. Postinfection (pneumonia, oesophageal perforation, peritonitis, subphrenic abscess, mediastinitis).
2. Postoperative (pneumonectomy, lobectomy, oesophagectomy, thoracotomy).
3. Post-traumatic (including iatrogenic oesophageal perforations).

Bacteriology may show anaerobic bacteria, Gram-negatives, staphylococcus, streptococcus and opportunistic infections in immunodepressed patients. The diagnosis is confirmed by chest X-rays and thoracocentesis.

Management of empyema must include antibiotic treatment, drainage of pus, lung re-expansion, treatment of primary causes, respiratory support if necessary, nutritional care and treatment of complications. Surgical options available are: tube thoracotomy, open thoracotomy, decortication, muscle transplants, space sterilisation and thoracoplasty.

Postresectional bronchopleural fistula

This is usually due to surgical trauma, ischaemia of the bronchial stump and/or poor technique, leading to local necrosis, infection and air-leak. The clinical signs start 1–2 weeks after the pulmonary resection. Massive expectoration of haemoserous or brown fluid with a decreased fluid level on the chest X-rays are characteristic of big fistulae. Sometimes these signs present early in the postoperative period and are usually predisposed to by poor surgical technique. The postpneumonectomy space becomes contaminated and eventually an empyema develops. The contralateral lung may get contaminated by overspilling fluid.

Treatment of this situation includes: drainage of the contaminated fluid with a fairly big chest drain, washouts of the cavity, antibiotics, oxygen, nutritional support, rib resection and open thoracotomy.

Further management is based on obliteration of the fistula through cauterisation, surgical glue or direct surgical repair.

Postpneumonectomy space

Management of drains is directed at maintaining the trachea central and expanding all remaining lung. Bleeding over 200 ml/hour for four consecutive hours, or more than 500 ml in any hour are indications for reopening.

Mediastinal shift of a massive degree and cardiac prolapse can cause a picture very like a massive pulmonary embolism or myocardial infarction. Mediastinal shift from unwise suction on the tube can quickly be corrected by releasing the drain to air. A cardiac prolapse must be treated by exploration and the return of the heart to the pericardium, which should then be made sufficiently competent to contain the heart reliably, or opened fully.

Septic shock

The term 'septic shock' refers to the association of the clinical features of cardiovascular failure with the presence of micro-organisms. However, it is not always possible to identify the causative organism, and the clinical features differ from shock caused by, for example, acute myocardial failure.

Sepsis is infection with various microorganisms, usually associated with systemic toxicity or fever.

Bacteraemia is the presence of demonstrable microorganisms in the blood.

Endotoxaemia is the clinical syndrome associated with infections resulting in various systemic manifestations (see below).

Septic shock is the condition of cardiovascular collapse due principally or exclusively to septicaemia; the result of an infective process that subsequently becomes systemic, bacteria or bacterial products entering the bloodstream, affecting the rest of the body. Primary sites are usually the lungs, the urinary tract, or intra-abdominal catastrophes such as bowel perforation. The features of septicaemia and septic shock are the same in all circumstances and are not related to the nature of the infecting organism.

Aetiological agents

Any organism may cause septicaemia, and in immunocompromised patients normal commensals or non-pathogenic organisms may do so. The most commonly encountered group of organisms are Gram-negative aerobic bacilli such as *E. coli* and, therefore, early antibiotic therapy is geared towards them. Blood culture must form the logical basis for therapy but unfortunately an organism is isolated in less than half of the patients.

Pathophysiology

Endotoxin is now known to be a portion of the bacterial cell membrane termed the lipid-A portion; levels in patients with septic shock are high, although the absolute level does not correlate with the severity.

Endotoxin activates many mediators of the inflammatory response: the prostaglandins, histamine and the kinin system and the complement and clotting cascades, and it produces endothelial damage, with precapillary vasoconstriction. Damage to the leucocyte with free radicals of oxygen also occurs.

Onset

Septic shock may occur quite rapidly, following surgical manipulation of an infected focus producing a sudden release of bacteria and endotoxin into the circulation. However, the onset may be insidious, with slow deterioration over several days. As a result, since the patient may be peripherally warm, appear pink and give a general appearance of not being particularly ill, it may be easy to miss the diagnosis and a high index of suspicion is essential.

Multi-organ involvement

Impaired cerebral function produces confusion, disorientation and depressed conscious levels.

Renal failure complicating septicaemia may occur despite satisfactory fluid balance and maintenance of adequate perfusion pressures of the kidney. In these circumstances it has been demonstrated that a form of glomerular nephritis occurs, possibly related to immune complex formation or to complement or other mediator-activated damage. Also, the patients may suffer acute tubular necrosis from hypoperfusion of the kidneys.

Respiratory involvement is associated with diffuse pulmonary oedema with infiltrates on chest X-ray, and progressive hypoxia.

Poor prognostic signs

- coagulation abnormalities
- granulocytopenia/thrombocytopenia
- no febrile response in first 24 hours
- age extremes, particularly the elderly
- development of secondary infection
- secondary organ involvement
- corticosteroid therapy (see below).

Mortality

Mortality is approximately 30%, irrespective of the aetiology. With the onset of secondary organ failure, mortality rates rise significantly – with either renal or respiratory failure, in excess of 75%.

Specific management

Management comprises eradication of the septic focus, drainage of intra-abdominal or other foci, re-exploration of cavities should the condition not improve and the use of appropriate antibiotics. Inappropriate antibiotic therapy has been shown to be associated with a higher mortality. Microbiological vigilance is essential and blood cultures should be taken at the slightest suspicion of sepsis, even in the absence of pyrexia.

Anaesthesia in thoracic surgery

Anaesthetic drugs

The pharmaceutical armamentarium required for thoracic anaesthesia differs little from that for other major surgery. The four tenets – anaesthesia, apnoea, muscle relaxation and analgesia – can be achieved nowadays, in general, by drugs with specific activity and minimal unwanted side-effects.

Three specific considerations may need to be anticipated.

1. Coexistent cardiac and/or pulmonary pathology.
2. Surgeon and anaesthetist may have to share or compete for the airway.
3. Drugs may affect:
   (a) pulmonary circulation;
   (b) hypoxic pulmonary vasoconstriction.

Induction agents

Most commonly-used induction agents produce a degree of cardiorespiratory depression which, in the compromised, may precipitate fatal complications. Although barbiturates, in the absence of known contraindications, are suitable for the fit (American Society of Anesthesiologists grades 1 and 2), agents such as etomidate or high-dose opioids are more suitable for the ill (ASA 3, 4 and 5).

Maintenance of anaesthesia

Non-flammable volatile agents remain the main agents for maintenance of anaesthesia, ensuring hypnosis and facilitating haemodynamic and circulatory manipulations. In small doses their use is not associated with the abolition of hypoxic pulmonary vasoconstriction, a natural protective mechanism that leads to the diversion of blood from areas of low ventilation and militates against the development of shunting; large doses may do so. Nitrous oxide is associated with an increase in pulmonary arterial pressure; its use is contraindicated in those with pulmonary hypertension or dysfunction of the right heart.

Intravenous anaesthesia

Competition for the airway by surgeon and anaesthetist, as for instance during bronchoscopy or tracheobronchial surgery, may necessitate the use of intravenous drugs to prevent awareness and to suppress reflexes because volatile agents may be difficult to administer. Several of the traditionally-used induction agents can be used, e.g. methohexitone, etomidate and propofol. Possible complications include cardiorespiratory depression and awareness.

Muscle relaxation

Muscle activity rarely prevents surgical access. Adequate access is usually attainable with bony retraction. Muscle-relaxant drugs facilitate the conduct of anaesthesia (tracheal intubation, institution and maintenance of positive pressure ventilation, suppression of diaphragmatic contraction).

Myaesthenia gravis

This is an uncommon autoimmune condition that results from a deficiency in the bioavailability of acetylcholine at the muscle end-plate. The autoimmune process appears to affect the number of postsynaptic acetylcholine receptors. It is often, though not exclusively, associated with pathology of the thymus gland. Females are more commonly afflicted; pregnancy or menstruation may result in deterioration. Usual presenting symptoms relate to easy fatiguability of muscle groups, notably ocular and bulbar muscle weakness, manifest in early stages as intermittent ptosis and palatal speech. The clinical classification (after Osserman and Genkins) may be used to stage the disease and define the severity of the disability. Psychological problems may be compounded by failure in diagnosis, organic pathology, therapy, and a restricted life-style. Aspiration pneumonia and respiratory failure are two associated life-threatening conditions that may result from disease progression or be precipitated by intercurrent illness, therapy, poor drug compliance, or anaesthesia and surgery. A similar disease, the rare Eaton-Lambert syndrome, is associated with bronchogenic malignancy.

Treatment

Aims are to improve the availability of acetylcholine at the muscle end-plate by suppressing cholinesterase activity with anticholinesterase drugs (e.g. pyridostigmine) and reducing autoimmune activity with steroids and immunosuppressant agents (e.g. azothioprine). Plasmapheresis may be indicated as a short-term therapeutic measure in extreme cases. Problems with regimes are common and can be difficult to differentiate from effects of the primary pathology. In some cases it may be necessary to stop all treatment and provide supportive artificial ventilation until the cause of deterioration can be elucidated and the patient restabilised.

Surgery and anaesthesia

Thymectomy by trans-sternal dissection, or surgery for concurrent illness, may be indicated. Extreme sensitivity to non-depolarisisng muscle-relaxant drugs is characteristic. These drugs should be avoided by using local and regional anaesthestic techniques, where possible, for surgery. In occasional situations, where muscle relaxation may be regarded as essential, e.g. tracheal intubation, depolarising agents (e.g. suxamethonium) can be used, although a degree of resistance to their activity may occur. The cautious use of newer, short-acting, muscle relaxants (e.g. vecuronium or atracurium, in part de-activated and degraded by a mechanism independent of acetylocholine – the Hoffman reaction) have been advocated, but experience of their use by specialists is limited and not definitive.

Intensive therapy

Bulbar incoordination, muscular fatigue, infection, surgery, sensitivity to analgesics, inadequate therapy, relative overdose and therapeutic desensitisation are situations that may precipitate respiratory dysfunction of sufficient severity to require intensive therapeutic support and artificial ventilation. Diagnostic difficulty may be encountered because both overdosage and underdosage of anticholinesterases may present as neuromuscular paralysis, the so-called cholinergic and myasthenic crises. Indications for which is the cause may be found by looking for signs of the muscarinic overactivity of acetylcholine (cholinergic crisis: lacrimation, sweating, miosis) and a trial of edrophonium (a short-acting anticholinesterase: cholinergic crises exacerbated/myasthenic crises improved).

Lung transplantation

Sufferers of chronic, non-malignant, progressive, pulmonary conditions with a fatal prognosis may benefit from lung transplantation. There is now reported experience of three forms of lung transplant surgery in which consistent success, in selected cases, has been achieved.

1. Heart and lung transplantation.
2. Bilateral lung transplantation.
3. Isolated lung transplantation.

Which of these is suitable depends on the pathophysiological state. Those most severely affected by cardiopulmonary disease generally require heart and lung transplantation; those with severe bilateral pulmonary disease, e.g. inflammatory or emphysematous disease, may be suitable recipients for bilateral lung transplantation. Certain diffuse and bilateral conditions, particularly alveolar fibroses with only mild aberrations of right ventricular function and moderate pulmonary hypertension, are suitable for orthotopic, isolated lung transplantation because the pathophysiology is such that the transplanted lung is favoured by not only being ventilated, but also perfused, in preference to the remaining, natural and diseased lung. Surgical and pharmacological care of the anastomoses between the donor's and recipient's airways are of the utmost importance.

Anaesthesia

Requirements of cases undergoing transplant operations (1) and (2) above are similar to those used routinely for surgery requiring cardiopulmonary bypass techniques. Early, successful experience has demonstrated that the operative requirements for isolated lung transplantation (3) are similar to those employed for major thoracic surgery, and are based on those evolved for one-lung anaesthesia. Lung separation is achieved either with double-lumen endobronchial tubes or by selective use of bronchial blockers. Problems may occur at certain operative points: if not controlled by first-line measures, partial cardiopulmonary bypass using the femoral vessels for vascular access may need to be instituted. The danger points are:

1. The induction of anaesthesia (cardiorespiratory collapse).
2. The onset of one-lung ventilation (respiratory failure).
3. Clamping and ligation of the pulmonary artery prior to pneumonectomy of the recipient.
4. Perfusion of donor lung (shunt, hypoxaemia).

Anaesthetic drugs favoured are those with stable pharmacological profiles in terms of their function on heart and lungs. Etomidate, short-acting opioids, and the new generation muscle relaxants are currently most suitable. Nitrous oxide should be eschewed and patients ventilated, during the operation and afterwards, with oxygen-enriched air.

Postoperative management

Postoperatively, in intensive care, the aim should be to withdraw patients from artificial ventilatory support as soon as criteria for weaning are met. Inotropic support is a valuable adjunct to preserving renal function because rigid fluid management is necessary to prevent interstitial pulmonary water accumulation. In those cases where omentum has been used to preserve airway anastomoses, some days of gastrointestinal disturbance may result from laparotomy. Steroids are not used routinely for immunosuppression until three weeks after operation, unless warranted for the management of acute rejection.

Postoperative pain relief for thoracic surgery

Four routes for nociceptive afferents from the thorax and its contents are recognised. These are the sympathetic chain, the intercostal nerves, the phrenic and vagus nerves. Other routes of lesser import are postulated and pain may pass centrally via more than one route: for example, from the parietal pleura it is mainly transmitted in intercostal nerves, but from the diaphragm it is mediated via the phrenic nerves, and from the mediastinum by the vagi.

Physiology

Pain is distressing, demoralising, and restricts activity. The inhibition of involuntary activity, such as breathing, is innately harmful. Operations differ quantitatively in painfulness, perhaps depending on how much muscle is cut, e.g. thoracotomy is worse than mediastinotomy. Pain produces a restrictive pattern of ventilation, with a fall in functional residual capacity due to diaphragmatic splinting, decreased pulmonary compliance, poor inspiratory effort, and failure to cough. This may lead to alveolar collapse, pulmonary atelectasis, ventilation and perfusion inequalities and shunting, of sufficient severity to produce hypoxaemia. Prophylaxis is best achieved with deep breathing, coughing, and physiotherapy, and pain relief is necessary to facilitate these. In those who have undergone abdominal surgery, effective analgesia results in functional improvement.

Analgesia

For the achievement of any degree of comfort in the acute phase after cardiothoracic surgery, powerful centrally-acting drugs are necessary. In clinical practice this can only be achieved with opioids and opiates. These can be administered sublingually, intramuscularly, extradurally or intraspinally, but the most certain is intravenously. The major complication of these drugs is respiratory depression. Patients in whom pain may precipitate respiratory failure may beneficially be maintained on a ventilator until the pain of acute injury is beginning to wear off.

Intercostal nerve block, including cryotherapy, can be done at surgery. More popular are local anaesthetic blocks which can be prolonged via strategically-placed catheters in the extradural or paravertebral space, or intercostally close to the angle of the rib. In general, the closer blockade is to the neuraxis, the greater its efficacy and the more extensive its nature, but the complication rate is more frequent. Some of these blocks will also affect the sympathetic chain with hypotension. Even with these techniques, patients may suffer acute distress by pathways not amenable to local anaesthetic blockade.

Pleural effusions in intensive care

Each pleura is a potential space lined by mesothelial membrane covering lungs and chest wall, which are kept together by the surface tension of the serous fluid, despite the subatmospheric pressure between lungs and chest wall. Up to 10 litres of fluid a day may move across the normal pleural space.

Pleural effusions may be classified into exudates (associated with inflammation of the pleura and with a protein content higher than 30 g/litre) and transudates (associated with hydrodynamic problems, usually heart failure).

The main causes of *exudates* are:
- malignant disease
- infection
- pulmonary infarction
- subphrenic/hepatic abscesses
- trauma
- post-myocardial infarction
- post-cardiotomy syndromes.

Transudates are predominantly produced by:
- heart failure
- cirrhosis of the liver
- nephrotic syndrome
- constrictive pericarditis
- hypoproteinaemia
- peritoneal dialysis.

Pleural effusions can alter pulmonary function by compression, especially when the lungs are diseased. They present with breathlessness, pleuritic pain, hypomotility of the chest, hyperventilation and bronchial breathing. The main investigations are:

1. *Plain X-rays* (particularly useful in intubated and ventilated patients whose clinical signs may be minimal). If it is possible to take the film in the upright position, 300–400 ml of fluid can be detected occluding the phrenic angle. Bigger effusions may cause 'white lungs'. If the X-ray is taken in a supine position, as much as 1000 ml of fluid may merely show a general haziness of the hemithorax, sometimes detected only by comparing the opacities of both sides.
2. *Ultrasound,* which is helpful when a directed thoracocentesis is to be performed.
3. *Aspiration and pleural biopsy.* The fluid must be analysed for:
   (a) colour (cloudy in exudates; bloody in malignant effusions, trauma and pulmonary infarction; milky in chylothorax; purulent in empyema);
   (b) glucose (less than 3 mmol/litre in infection and malignancy);
   (c) amylase (high in pancreatitis);
   (d) cytology;
   (e) bacteriology;
   (f) histopathology.

The initial object is to diagnose the underlying condition by fluid aspiration and biopsy. If the effusion recurs after two aspirations, thoracoscopy and biopsy should be considered if the diagnosis is not clear. Otherwise, recurrent effusions might need tube drainage, talc pleurodesis, pleurectomy or pleuroperitoneal shunt, in very selected cases.

Following cardiac surgery, pleural effusions in the left side are quite common, especially when the left internal mammary artery has been mobilised for grafting. When the pleura has been opened inadvertently, a large collection of blood and cardioplegic solution can occur. Intrapleural bleeding may be the cause of postoperative hypovolaemia. Late pleural effusions may be caused by a post-cardiotomy syndrome.

Following pulmonary resection, the main cause of pleural effusion is bleeding. Late effusions may represent the onset of an empyema. Early pleural effusions after oesophagoscopy and/or dilatation may represent oesophageal perforation.

Acute mediastinal syndromes

The mediastinum is bounded by the sternum anteriorly, the spine posteriorly, the diaphragm inferiorly, the pleural cavities on either side, and continues with the neck superiorly. It contains the heart, great vessels, oesophagus, trachea, thymus, nerves and lymph nodes.

Mediastinitis

Mediastinitis may be secondary to another life-threatening condition, e.g. perforation or anastomotic leakage of the oesophagus, penetrating wounds of the chest or postoperative contamination. Clinical features include:

- severe deterioration
- chest pain
- rigors
- pyrexia
- dyspnoea
- cyanosis
- dysphagia.

The treatment is basically the correction of the primary condition, with supportive sedation, oxygen, antibiotics and early surgical drainage.

Mediastinal emphysema

The presence of air in the mediastinum occurs with perforation of the oesophagus or central airways, or with positive pressure ventilation and in some cases is spontaneous and unexplained. Physical signs are:

- substernal pain
- crepitus in the neck
- cardiac 'crunch' on auscultation (Hamman's sign)
- dyspnoea
- venous engorgement.

Chest X-rays reveal the presence of mediastinal air and studies should be directed to find the cause, oesophageal perforation being one of the most serious. Treatment is directed towards the underlying cause.

Superior vena caval syndrome

This results from obstruction of the superior vena cava. The main clinical features are:

- oedema of head, neck, arms and chest
- dilated venous collaterals in the chest wall
- cyanosis
- neurological impairment (occasionally).

Some causes are malignancies (lung, thyroid, thymus), idiopathic mediastinal fibrosis, mediastinal goitre and aortic arch diseases. Diagnosis is achieved by chest X-rays, bronchoscopy, CT scan and venous angiography. The majority of patients have inoperable tumours which can be palliated by radiotherapy, providing venous decompression.

Blood transfusion in thoracic surgery

Transfusion of blood or its products is not without hazard, and should not be undertaken lightly, especially in those cases of pneumonectomy with previous cardiac disease in whom fluid overload may be lethal.

Transfusion may be done with whole blood or appropriate blood components.

Whole blood

Every 500 ml of anticoagulated blood contains approximately 440 ml of donor's blood and 60 ml of citrate phosphate dextrose. Blood should be kept at 4–6°C and must be rejected if the expiry date is passed. Whole blood is used in cases of major bleeding, especially if the postoperative losses reach 500–1000 ml over the first 6–8 hours after the operation. If the losses are greater than that, a decision should be made between treatment of clotting defects or surgical re-exploration.

Plasma-reduced blood

This is whole blood with its plasma and anticoagulant removed. The haematocrit is approximately 60%. Its main use is red cell replacement in patients with pulmonary, hepatic, renal or cardiac disease, in whom fluid overload must be avoided.

Concentrated red cells

In this preparation the haematocrit is about 70%. It is used in the same circumstances as is plasma-reduced blood.

Leucocyte-depleted blood

The leucocytes are removed from the blood in this preparation. It is indicated in cases of non-haemolytic febrile transfusion reaction in patients with previous transfusions who have positive antibodies (leucocyte-specific or histocompatibility locus antigen (HLA) antibodies).

Platelets

These are used with thrombocytopenia lower than 10×10^9/litre, especially if there is any haematological malignancy, chemotherapy, irradiation or active bleeding. It is also indicated in patients with previous platelet defect, either congenital or secondary to massive transfusions. The dose is usually 4–10 units.

Granulocytes

The main use of this preparation is in patients with severe leucopenia ($< 0.5 \times 10^9$/litre) with evidence of active pulmonary infection refractory to antibiotic treatment. Its use is very rare and must be haematologically mandatory, since it can cause serious pulmonary damage.

Fresh frozen plasma

In 200 ml all the coagulation factors are present. It is administered in cases of:

- congenital deficiency of factors V and XI
- haemophiliacs awaiting specific transfusion but bleeding seriously
- disseminated intravascular coagulation
- severe hepatic disease
- vitamin K deficiency
- overdose of oral anticoagulants
- massive transfusions
- non-surgical bleeding after cardiopulmonary bypass.

The dose is usually 10–15 ml/kg, or 3–6 units.

Cryoprecipitate

The volume is around 80 ml. The main use is in deficiency of factor VIII – either congenital or acquired (trauma, surgery) – or in cases of severe infection with pulmonary involvement in which fibronectin, which is present in cryoprecipitate, should be given. The dose is 6 to 12 packs.

Albumin

There are two preparations: plasma protein factor (PPF) and albumin. The most common uses are in hypovolaemia and protein depletion but its routine use has been questioned because of its cost and the effect on the lung if previous disease has been present.

Plasma substitutes

These are solutions of macromolecules with some plasma-like properties (colloid osmotic pressure, viscosity). They do not contain haemoglobin, antibodies or clotting factors; their main use is replacement of volume. The main examples are: dextran solutions (which should be avoided in cases of bleeding, since they can dilute clotting factors) and Hespan.

Some *complications* of transfusions are:

- febrile reactions
- circulatory overload
- haemolysis
- air embolism
- allergy
- infection due to bacterial contamination
- donor's transmitted infection (syphilis, hepatitis B, AIDS).

Postoperative nursing care of the thoracic surgical patient

The main aim of postoperative care is to prevent complications.

The early stages

Care starts before the patient's return from theatre by preparing the bed space. A clean, warm bed, appropriately folded, is made ready. In addition:

1. Oxygen supply checked and mask at hand.
2. Wall suction unit cleared and checked, adequate tubing connected and a good supply of suction catheters of varying sizes installed.
3. Portable suction unit available in the room.
4. Cardiac monitor and accessories available and checked.
5. Set of tubing clamps, drip stand, drainage-bottle holder available.
6. Postoperative intensive care chart, thermometers and syphgmomanometer at hand.

Return from theatre

On transfer from trolley to bed the pleural drains are securely clamped, and unclamped as the patient is settled into his bed, checking that they are not displaced or disconnected. The surgical wound is inspected (without disturbing the dressing) for any seepage of blood, haematoma, or subcutaneous emphysema.

Baseline observations of pulse, apex, blood pressure and respirations are monitored; the backrest and pillows are arranged to allow a sitting position and the drains are secured accordingly.

Maintaining adequate lung function

The patient is positioned upright as soon as possible and deep breathing and coughing encouraged. Observations of the trend of breathing, maintenance of a clear airway and administration of oxygen (35–40% at 8–12 litres) are necessary until the patient can manage with room air.

Pain control and relief of anxiety

Reassurance that the operation is completed and that the patient is back in bed is complemented by prescribed analgesia. This is usually given intravenously via a syringe pump (morphine 50 mg with 50 ml saline, at between 1–2 ml/h. Deep breathing and coughing are encouraged. Too much analgesia can depress the respiratory centre and cough reflex but too little allows pain to inhibit respiratory and coughing movements.

Explanation of the equipment and procedures being carried out decreases the patient's anxiety and gains his co-operation.

Pleural drains

In the pneumonectomy patient drains are left on free drainage without suction and the seal is broken hourly to centralise the mediastinum.

In lobectomies and other thoracic surgical patients, the drains are attached to low suction (10–20 mmHg) and milked regularly.

The amount of drainage and air are recorded half-hourly, increasing to hourly; excessive amounts are promptly reported.

A chest radiograph is performed on the evening of surgery and again the following morning. Continuous ECG monitoring allows half-hourly to hourly rates and changes of rhythm to be reported. Blood pressure is recorded half-hourly. Urinary output, nausea, vomiting and abdominal distension are also noted.

Hydration

Prescribed intravenous fluids, e.g. dextrose–saline 70–100 ml/h, are administered, maintaining a patent line at all times and observing the site of entry for leakage, swelling, redness and discomfort.

Mouth toilet/wash is performed 2-hourly until the patient commences oral intake, which is usually the following morning.

Antibiotics are generally given intravenously 6-hourly until the patient commences oral intake.

Movement

Early after operation, whilst in bed, encouragement is given to move arms and legs. Pressure areas are checked and treated 2-hourly, turning the patient, except following a pneumonectomy when the patient is lifted to avoid mediastinal shift.

During this immobile period calcium–heparin is given sub-cutaneously 5000 units b.d.

The dressings are checked regularly but left intact and only moved if necessary. The patient is encouraged to hold the wound area when coughing. To make the patient more comfortable, refreshed and more settled, a bed-bath is given on the evening of surgery and again the following morning.

Paediatric pulmonary disease

Respiratory failure in the neonate

Neonates differ physiologically from adults and older children, being more susceptible to critical illness. The physiological changes associated with birth are enormous and are not complete for some time after birth, during which the neonate may revert to a fetal circulatory pattern.

Neonates respond to varied pathological processes with a limited number of physical signs, so that respiratory problems may reflect many differing respiratory or non-respiratory diseases. The decision to provide respiratory support may sometimes be made on clinical grounds despite current relatively normal blood gases.

Clinically, a neonate has 'respiratory distress' if two or more of the following signs are present:

- tachypnoea (respiratory rate over 70)
- cyanosis
- intractable or repeated apnoea
- retraction of chest wall on inspiration.

There may be associated signs such as restlessness, difficulty in feeding, flaring of nostrils or grunting on expiration. Clinical judgement may be supported by arterial blood gas analysis showing hypoxaemia and/or ventilatory failure.

Pulmonary causes of respiratory failure

Generally it is unusual for respiratory failure to arise solely from postnatal events. A review of the pre- and perinatal history (particularly gestational age) will often provide much useful information.

Physiological background

Neonates have less respiratory reserve than adults and older children. Compared with adults they have a higher metabolic rate

282

and oxygen consumption, and alveolar ventilation is increased twofold.

The ribs are more horizontal and the intercostal muscles weak, making the chest wall very compliant and not able to maintain stability and oppose the action of the diaphragm (particularly in REM sleep when the intercostals are centrally inhibited). Thus, the functional residual capacity (FRC) – the volume of gas left in the lung at the end of a normal breath (and the buffer against hypoxia) – is low, particularly in proportion to alveolar ventilation.

The closing volume is high and may exceed the FRC. This means that, in normal breathing, air trapping may occur and give rise to ventilation–perfusion imbalance; this is probably why the normal neonatal Pao_2 is only 9.5–10 kPa in air. As the FRC reservoir of intrapulmonary gas is low, neonates are rapidly affected by changes in inspired gas concentrations.

With a highly compliant chest wall, increase in ventilation must be achieved largely by an increase in rate rather than tidal volume. However, in neonates the diaphragm becomes fatigued. Only 30% of diaphragmatic muscle fibres are type 1 (fatigue resistant, slow twitch) and the proportion is even lower in premature neonates. The percentage increases to that of the adult (50–55%) over the first year or so. Neonates may thus become exhausted and deteriorate rapidly if the work of breathing is increased, so they must be carefully watched.

The airway has a much smaller lumen and is more easily compromised by small reductions in diameter caused, for example, by inflammatory changes. Neonates are obligate nasal breathers and cannot compensate for blocked nasal passages by mouth breathing.

The list of causes of neonatal respiratory failure given in Table 6.1 is by no means exhaustive but serves to illustrate the variety of conditions which may give rise to, or present as, respiratory failure. Treatment should not only be aimed at the effect (respiratory failure) but also the cause.

Effects of respiratory failure

Pulmonary arteriolar smooth muscle is present in larger amounts in neonates than adults, and contracts in the presence of hypoxia, hypercapnia and acidaemia, increasing pulmonary vascular resistance, and encouraging right-to-left shunting through the foramen ovale and ductus arteriosus. Hence hypoxia and acidosis are worsened, further raising pulmonary vascular resistance, and a vicious circle develops.

Table 6.1 Some causes of respiratory failure in neonates

CNS (diminished respiratory effort)
  prematurity: recurrent apnoeas and periodic breathing
  convulsions: may manifest as apnoeas
  septicaemias
  metabolic problems: hypocalcaemia and other electrolyte disturbances,
    hypoglycaemia and metabolic acidosis
  drugs (including maternal and anaesthetic drugs)
  intracranial haemorrhage
  hypothermia

Intrapulmonary
  respiratory distress syndrome (RDS) (or hyaline membrane disease)
  infection
  aspiration of meconium
  transient tachypnoea of the newborn (residual pulmonary interstitial fluid)

Intrathoracic obstruction
  pneumothorax
  diaphragmatic hernia
  intrathoracic mass or cyst

Secondary to congenital heart disease
  large left-to-right shunts (e.g. PDA or VSD)
  aortic stenosis and other left-heart obstructions causing pulmonary oedema (see
    Section III)

Other
  obstruction of airways (e.g. choanal atresia, vascular ring)
  severe acute loss of blood
  diaphragmatic splinting (e.g. distension of bowel, and after repair of
    exomphalos)

In the neonate, the cardiovascular response to acute hypoxia differs from that seen in adults. Rather than tachycardia and hypertension, bradycardia and hypotension may occur. Flow of blood to the kidneys and extremities is reduced. Sweating does not occur.

Principles of treatment

It is important to maintain oxygenation to prevent persistent fetal circulation, while treating the underlying cause. In some disorders, such as pneumothorax, a prompt diagnosis is life saving, but if initially undetermined, general supportive measures for the relief of hypoxia are instituted until the correct diagnosis becomes clear.

1. Maintain oxygenation by increasing F_{IO_2}.
2. Physiotherapy.

3. Pulmonary vasodilators (e.g. prostacyclin, tolazoline, nitrog-lycerine).
4. Maintain systemic circulation with volume expanders and inotropes if necessary. (Note that dobutamine tends to reduce neonatal pulmonary vascular resistance whereas dopamine may increase it.)
5. Oral feeding should be replaced with parenteral nutrition at an early stage as feeding difficulties cause risk from abdominal distension, regurgitation and aspiration.
6. Maintain temperature: hypothermia markedly increases oxygen consumption and CO_2 production from the increased metabolic rate of shivering.
7. Correction of acidosis: repeated doses of bicarbonate may be harmful. Severe respiratory acidosis is best dealt with by treating the cause (hypercapnia) by improving ventilation, or instituting artificial ventilation. (Note that artificially-fed neonates often have a mild metabolic acidosis, but arterial pH < 7.18 should be treated.)
8. CPAP (constant distending pressure) helps maintain FRC by maintaining patency of airways and alveoli during expiration and often, particularly in respiratory distress syndrome (RDS), reduces oxygen requirements.
9. Consider ventilation: ventilator-induced respiratory alkalosis will help reduce PVR.

Monitoring and assessment

Repeated observation by an expert (preferably the same), should detect increasing respiratory distress or the onset of fatigue. Bedside observation of respiratory rate and the presence, for example, of retractions, is of more immediate value than measurements of respiratory mechanics which are of limited value in the acute situation and are in any case difficult and unreliable in neonates.

Blood gas analysis – a trend is more useful than individual measurements, which may be unreliable, especially if sampling was difficult. Continuous transcutaneous gas analysis is very useful but may be unreliable in poorly-perfused neonates. Pulse oximetry is increasingly used but is less useful in detecting neonatal hypoxia. In babies with a patent ductus arteriosus it should be remembered that the right arm is supplied with preductal blood.

Thoracic auscultation is of limited value in the neonate, and may be misleading. Its reliability is probably limited to establishing the presence of symmetrical breath sounds.

Chest X-rays are invaluable, especially if of sufficiently consistent quality to enable valid comparison to be made between films.

Transillumination of the thorax with a powerful fibreoptic light source may detect pneumothorax in an emergency in neonates. Bilateral pneumothoraces, however, may be missed.

Examination of the airway by laryngoscopy or bronchoscopy may be necessary to confirm suspected narrowing of the airways.

Complications of therapy which are specific to neonates

Retrolental fibroplasia

High arterial oxygen concentrations have a vasoconstrictive effect on the retinal arteries of neonates. While occasional, very short periods of hyperoxia are probably harmless, the precise levels and duration of hyperoxia causing retrolental hyperplasia are not known and other causative factors are thought to exist. It is generally recommended that the Pao_2 be kept below 80 mmHg (10.6 kPa).

Bronchopulmonary dysplasia (BPD)

Artificially ventilated neonates may develop chronic ventilatory insufficiency. Factors involved include high peak ventilatory pressures (which may be minimised by sedation and muscle-relaxants to prevent straining) and direct pulmonary oxygen toxicity. There is damage to the bronchial walls leading to an obstructive emphysema which is usually diffuse but may be localised. As the BPD progresses, pulmonary hypertension and cor pulmonale may develop, and as lung damage continues, high ventilatory pressures and concentrations of inspired oxygen are necessary, which in themselves worsen matters.

Thoracic problems in the neonate

Respiratory distress syndrome (RDS; hyaline membrane disease)

This occurs in nearly 1% of all births and is the commonest cause of neonatal death. It is due to a relative deficiency of pulmonary surfactant, a surface-active material which normally maintains alveolar stability. Factors commonly found on review of the history include prematurity, maternal diabetes and antepartum haemorrhage.

An antenatal prediction of pulmonary maturity may be made by amniotic fluid analysis for lecithin and sphyngomyelin. Adequate surfactant is indicated by a lecithin:sphyngomyelin ratio of 2 or more and is normally achieved by the 35th week of gestation. Intra-uterine stress, or its simulation with maternally administered steroids, may induce early production of surfactant and at least partly explains why some premature infants escape RDS.

Postnatally, production of surfactant is inhibited by hypoxia and acidosis. The pulmonary capillaries leak into the alveoli, and fibrinous membranes are formed in the alveoli. These hyaline membranes are an incidental finding and are not the basic cause of the pulmonary problems.

The unstable, fluid-containing alveoli prevent the formation of an FRC, and the V/Q ratio is markedly unbalanced. The poorly-compliant lungs greatly increase the work of breathing. A transitional circulatory pattern may develop.

Clinical features

Immediately after birth no sign may be obvious, but features of respiratory distress are usually present by four hours. If signs develop after eight hours of life, a diagnosis other than RDS should be sought (although rarely older neonates and infants may develop adult RDS). Generally, the earlier the onset of symptoms, the more severe the course of the disease. Expiratory grunting is often the first sign, followed by retraction of ribs, tachypnoea, and other signs of respiratory failure. Auscultation usually just reveals an overall diminution of breath sounds, occasionally with bronchial breathing. Chest X-rays show diffuse granularity (the characteristic 'ground-glass appearance') due to widespread alveolar collapse. The more severe cases may also show an air bronchogram.

Management

The artificial instilling of surfactant, which has been performed experimentally, is not yet routine clinically. Management at present is directed towards allowing the natural production of surfactant by preventing hypoxia, maintaining a normal circulation and preventing acidosis. In milder cases, elevation of FIO_2 may suffice to maintain arterial oxygen partial pressure within the range 8–10 kPa. If this fails, early CPAP is advised, and may reduce the later necessity for IPPV. As neonates are obligate nasal breathers, CPAP may be applied by nasal prongs, initially at about

4–5 cmH$_2$O up to 10 cmH$_2$O if necessary. IPPV is indicated if this fails to give an arterial Pao$_2$ > 6.5 kPa, a Pco$_2$ < 8.5 and pH > 7.2.

Emergencies

The most likely cause of a sudden deterioration is a pneumothorax or a mechanical ventilatory problem. Other causes of deterioration include development of transitional circulation, pulmonary haemorrhage, intraventricular haemorrhage, pneumonia and hypoglycaemia.

Transient tachypnoea of the newborn

A delay in the clearance of pulmonary fluid, particularly when delivery was by caesarean section, is probably responsible for this syndrome. It presents as a mild form of RDS with tachypnoea as the main sign, occasionally accompanied by slight rib retractions. Chest X-rays show reticular shadowing, sometimes with small effusions. Neonates rarely require more than a raised Fio$_2$, or CPAP, and the condition usually resolves in under three or four days. Some small infants may develop respiratory failure and require ventilation.

Diaphragmatic hernia

The incidence of this is about 1 in 3500 births. Most commonly, the abdominal viscera herniate through the left side of the diaphragm posterolaterally, through the foramen of Bochdalek. It is associated with gut malrotation in 40% of cases and congenital heart disease in over 10%. The associated respiratory failure is due both to compression and hypoplasia of the lung. The pulmonary hypoplasia will be more severe if herniation has occurred early in intrauterine life, and is a major prognostic factor.

Clinical features

The apex beat is displaced away from the affected side. The abdomen may appear scaphoid. On the affected side of the chest there may be audible bowel sounds as well as diminished breath sounds and reduced movement of the chest wall. Severe cases show signs of respiratory distress at birth and require immediate resuscitation. Diagnosis is confirmed by chest X-ray.

Management

Prior to surgery, avoid further distension of intrathoracic viscera. Do not ventilate with a mask but intubate immediately if ventilation is required. Pass a nasogastric tube and suck continuously or regularly every five minutes. The patient is usually best lying toward the affected side with the head of the cot slightly raised. Some centres have a policy of immediate operation whilst others have a short period of stabilisation prior to operation.

Babies with severely hypoplastic lungs may succumb rapidly despite all measures. Others in whom pulmonary compression is the problem recover quickly after operation. The third, intermediate, group with some hypoplasia may develop hypoxia and acidosis and require ventilatory support. High ventilatory pressures may be unavoidable to maintain oxygenation but are likely to lead to pulmonary damage and increase the risk of pneumothorax. Experimentally, extracorporeal oxygenation has been used in this situation.

Pneumothorax (on either side) and sudden reversion to transitional circulation are common urgent situations. The latter is common because the small pulmonary vascular bed has very labile tone. As well as a high F_{IO_2}, a pulmonary vasodilator, particularly tolazoline or prostacyclin, may be given by infusion.

Tracheosophageal fistula

Oesophageal atresia and tracheosophageal fistula are related conditions and have an incidence of 1 in 3000 live births. A simple fistula between trachea and oesophagus is relatively uncommon; diagnosis is not easy and is often only made after repeated chest infections later in infancy. Most commonly there is a blind upper oesophagus with a fistula from the lower trachea to the distal segment of the oesophagus. Antenatally, polyhydramnios is common, and about one-third of affected babies are born prematurely. About 50% of affected babies have an associated abnormality, usually gastrointestinal, cardiac or renal.

Clinical features

Saliva is seen dribbling from the mouth. There may be episodes of choking and cyanosis, particularly if the baby is unfortunate enough to be fed, when pulmonary aspiration may occur. It is not possible to pass a nasogastric tube and, if it has not coiled up, an X-ray showing its tip will thus show the length of the upper oesophageal pouch. Also, if there is a blind oesophagus and the X-ray shows air in the stomach, then the presence of a fistula is confirmed, as the air must have got to the stomach through the fistula.

Management

Prevent aspiration by witholding oral feeds and suctioning the oesophageal pouch. A double-lumen Replogle tube is best: low-pressure suction is applied to one channel whilst the other admits air to prevent the tube sticking to the side of the pouch. Gastro-oesophageal reflux is reduced by a head-up tilt of the cot. If aspiration is suspected then antibiotics and intensive physiotherapy should be instituted before operation.

Unless aspiration and subsequent pneumonitis have occurred it is unlikely that pre-operative ventilation will be necessary in a full-term baby. If intubation is required, do not paralyse the baby beforehand as that would necessitate 'bagging' with a mask and blowing gases through the fistula. Check with a stethoscope that the gases are flowing into both lungs and not into the stomach. If the stomach is being inflated then reposition the tube either by rotating it so that the bevel points in a different direction or by passing it a little further into the trachea.

After operation, ventilation is usually only required if there has been pre-operative aspiration, if the baby was premature and has developed RDS, or if necessitated by other congenital abnormalities. Occasionally, the oeosphagus is tight and the baby is paralysed and sedated to prevent straining and tension on the anastomosis. Sudden deterioration may be due to anastomostic breakdown. If the oesophageal defect is found to be too big, anastomosis is delayed and continuous upper-pouch suction must be employed, with magnetic elongation to facilitate future end-to-end anastomosis.

Aspiration of meconium

An asphyxiating fetus may pass meconium into the amniotic fluid and make gasping movements. Meconium is inhaled and results in chemical pneumonitis and plugging of airways. Areas of consolidation are interspersed with areas where a valve-like action of the plugs has resulted in air trapping and hyperinflation.

Clinical features

The meconium-stained newborn baby may be in respiratory failure at birth, and has irregular gasping respirations. In less severe cases tachypnoea is the main feature. The chest may appear hyper-inflated. The radiological appearance of coarse, widely-scattered densities may not appear for a day or two.

Management

To prevent further aspiration, the larynx is visualised immediately and any meconium is removed. Following intubation the trachea is washed out with saline, and the stomach aspirated to prevent further inhalation of meconium after a vomit.

General supportive care for respiratory failure is given as described elsewhere. There is often a poor response to simple administration of oxygen, indicating a considerable degree of shunting. It is not possible to distinguish meconium aspiration from pneumonia with certainty, and a 'septic screening' followed by antibiotics is advisable. The most important complications are pneumothorax and pneumomediastinum.

Pneumonia

Neonates are at risk of infection because of their immature immune systems. The infection may arise from infected amniotic fluid following prolonged rupture of the membranes, in which case signs are present soon after birth, or, uncommonly, from transplacental spread of viral infection. Other sources of infection are passage through an infected birth canal and cross-infection from other neonates. The commonest organisms involved are *E. coli*, streptococci and staphylococcus, with pseudomonas a potential risk to ventilated babies.

Diagnostic pointers include prolonged rupture of membranes, bad-smelling amniotic fluid or maternal vaginal discharge, or maternal fever prior to delivery. Deterioration during the course of any pulmonary disease may represent pneumonia. Invasive procedures, such as intubation, increase the risk.

Clinical features

Pneumonia is not always easy to diagnose, e.g. the difficulty of differentiating between pneumonia and meconium aspiration. X-ray appearances vary and may show bilateral or unilateral consolidation, diffuse mottling or haziness. The WBC count may be high or very low.

Management

As well as general supportive measures, it is advisable to start treatment with antibiotics as soon as pneumonia is suspected. A broad spectrum combination such as penicillin and gentamicin should be used while awaiting the results of cultures. Delay, particularly in treating group B haemolytic streptococcal infections, may be disastrous. Complications include empyema and pneumatocoeles (especially but not exclusively in staphylococcal infections).

Cystic pulmonary conditions in neonates

These may be congenital or acquired and are rare. They are mentioned because they are a cause of serious respiratory distress in neonates. Most cystic lesions are lobar emphysemas. Several aetiologies have been suggested for the congenital type. The bronchial cartilage may be deficient, causing collapse during expiration and air trapping, or obstruction may be caused by extrinsic pressure from abnormal vessels or enlarged lymph glands. Acquired lobar emphysema usually arises as a complication of RDS and its treatment, during which air is forced along perivascular spaces during ventilation. As increasing numbers of patients with severe RDS are surviving, most pulmonary cysts seen are of this type.

Clinical features

Symptoms may present at birth or may develop gradually. Signs are those of respiratory distress, with mediastinal shift as the affected lobe gets bigger. Although X-rays may appear superficially similar to a pneumothorax, or possibly even a diaphragmatic hernia, careful examination will show lung markings.

Management

Untreated congenital lobar emphysemas have a significant mortality and the lobe should be surgically excised, following which there is good recovery and minimal effect on pulmonary function in the long term. Surgery is urgent if there are signs of mediastinal shift. There is no place for needle aspiration. Occasionally, bronchoscopy will reveal a mucous plug obstructing the bronchial lumen which can be removed. Ventilation may be hazardous as it may cause further distension of the lobe. Acquired lobar emphysemas frequently resolve over a period of months without treatment. If, however, lung perfusion scans show absent perfusion of the affected lobe, or if the infant deteriorates clinically, then lobectomy is performed.

Other types of cystic lesion are seen rarely and cause respiratory distress, necessitating removal. Cystic adenomatoid malformations are initially full of fluid and need to be differentiated from solid mediastinal lesions such as neurofibromas, neuroblastomas or teratomas. As the fluid is absorbed, they become air filled and may resemble diaphragmatic hernias if a single X-ray, rather than a series, is examined.

Choanal atresia

While this is not strictly intrathoracic, it is, if bilateral, a life-threatening condition which, when recognised, is easily dealt with. Respiratory distress is present from birth, with marked retractions of the ribs and cyanosis. Babies are obligate nasal breathers and cannot breathe orally except when crying, which relieves the symptoms. A nasogastric tube cannot be passed through the nose. The obstruction is immediately relieved by the life-saving insertion of an oral airway which is held in place with adhesive tape, pending surgery.

Acute obstruction of upper airways in children

The development of upper airways obstruction in childhood (as opposed to neonates) is relatively uncommon in hospital practice, but not rare. In the community, mild forms are seen more frequently, usually in association with upper respiratory tract infections. We will deal with the problems encountered in hospital practice, in particular those seen on a general ITU.

Aetiology

There are three common causes of acute obstruction of upper airways in childhood:

1. Acute epiglottitis.
2. Croup, i.e. subglottic stenosis.
3. Foreign body.

The last cause (foreign body) is less commonly seen on an ITU than the other two, and is usually dealt with in the Accident and

Emergency department. This section will therefore discuss the first two causes of airways obstruction only.

Other less common aetiologies are occasionally encountered, and may present similar clinical findings. They include tumours affecting the upper airway, abscesses, and trauma. Fortunately these are rare.

Clinical features

The common features of epiglottitis and croup are related to the obstruction of the upper airways. Usually the first signs are non-specific and related to a preceding mild upper respiratory tract infection, with or without cough. The child then develops noisy breathing with both an inspiratory and expiratory stridor. This is in contradistinction to obstruction of lower airways, such as in asthma, when the child has predominantly expiratory obstruction. Associated with the stridor are two clinical signs, tracheal tug and inter- and subcostal recession, resulting from the thoracic boundaries being 'sucked' inward. This has the additional effect of adding considerably to the work of breathing. Indeed, the rapid onset of fatigue in these circumstances is often the factor precipitating intervention in the form of intubation.

These clinical findings are common to all causes of acute obstruction of the upper airways, and the differentiation between diseases usually depends on the other features of the individual disease.

Acute epiglottitis

This is an acute inflammation of the epiglottis and peri-epiglottic structures, usually confined to the supraglottic area. The true cords and structures below them are never directly involved and the inflamed area usually remains very localised. The resultant oedema in such a critical site may rapidly produce total obstruction of the airway.

The disease occurs throughout childhood with a peak incidence in the second year of life, and is often seasonal, although the actual season varies in different regions in the country.

The commonest causative organism isolated is *Haemophilus influenzae,* followed by various viruses, such as influenza and parainfluenza viruses. Diagnosis is clinical, and an organism is often not isolated from swabs or blood culture.

The disease usually begins suddenly, often progressing to severe obstruction in a matter of hours. The child often has preceding difficulty in swallowing, is toxic with a high fever, and lethargic.

They often adopt a characteristic posture, sitting up and leaning forward with the head held backwards and the chin thrust forward. Presumably this is an attempt to increase the patency of the upper airway, and the posture mimics the position of the head for intubation. The child is usually drooling saliva, as swallowing past the acutely inflamed epiglottis is painful. Cough is not a common feature.

Croup: subglottic stenosis

This disease is part of a more widespread infection of the respiratory tract, affecting not just the upper airways but extending through the bronchial tree. This is termed laryngo-tracheobronchitis and is a common infection in paediatric practice. A minority of patients with this infection develop obstruction at the site of the cricoid cartilage. Presumably the children who develop this have always had a narrower cricoid ring than the average, but under normal circumstances the lumen is adequate. Once infection occurs, the resultant inflammation and oedema reduce the lumen critically. As the cricoid is the only complete cartilage ring, oedema must encroach on the lumen of the trachea, and if this is already narrowed then very little swelling will produce stridor.

The most common organisms responsible are viral, in particular the respiratory syncytial virus, followed by the influenzal group. Bacterial infection almost never produces this picture. Seasonal variation occurs according to the peak incidences of the causative organism.

Croup tends to occur throughout childhood, especially in the second year of life. Severe airways obstruction is likewise seen in the younger child, and decreases as the cricoid grows, although it always remains the narrowest part of the airway, and its effect on airways resistance is related to the square of the radius (Poiseuille's equation).

The child with croup usually has a slower onset of disease than epiglottitis, has a productive cough, often 'barking' in nature, and may be unable to vocalise. The child is often restless, and is not toxic, with only a mild pyrexia. The onset of airways obstruction is less dramatic but both diseases may result in an exhausted patient, hypoxic with severe obstruction.

Management

The principal decision is the timing of intervention, i.e. intubation. Early, mild forms have been treated conservatively, with oxygen, humidification and observation. Steroids and nebulised adrenaline may reduce the amount of oedema. Steroids have had disappointing results, and may impair responses to infection. Nebulised adrenaline does shorten the average period of stridor in croup, possibly avoiding intubation in some patients. Its use in epiglottitis is not as clear, and at present cannot be recommended.

The usual factor precipitating intubation is the onset of fatigue with the development of type II failure (see p. 219). Any form of instrumentation of the upper airway may provoke intense laryngeal spasm, particularly in epiglottitis. Should intubation be required, examination under anaesthesia immediately beforehand is permissible. Examination of the upper airway is not advisable merely to establish the diagnosis of epiglottitis as the clinical manifestations are sufficient.

Anaesthesia is induced with 100% oxygen with halothane. Intravenous access, if not already *in situ,* is established prior to examination of the upper airway. Equipment must include a full range of tubes, laryngoscope and mini-tracheostomy and tracheostomy instruments. The appearance of the epiglottis in this condition bears little relationship to normal anatomy, as the structures are swollen and oedematous and 'cherry red'; the oedema is soft but, if the glottis can be located, intubation is not too difficult. It is our practice in epiglottitis to intubate orally and then to change this to a nasotracheal tube. We have never had to resort to tracheostomy in this condition.

In subglottic stenosis and croup the supraglottic area is normal and intubation through the cords presents no problem. However, the tube often sticks at the cricoid area and it may be necessary to resort to a much smaller diameter endotracheal tube than anticipated from the size of the child. Should the tube need to be changed to a smaller size, it is possible to hand ventilate with the tube just through the glottis. It is rare to need tracheostomy in the acute phase.

Epiglottitis usually settles within 48 hours with appropriate antibiotic therapy. A further examination under anaesthesia is carried out at this time and extubation is undertaken under anaesthesia. In subglottic stenosis the illness usually lasts 7–10 days and at extubation examination is carried out under anaesthesia. In this condition postextubation stridor is not uncommon as, on occasion, the presence of the tube perpetuates the oedema despite resolution of the infection. Under these circumstances tracheostomy may be required to avoid prolonged intubation through the narrowed segment.

Prognosis of both these conditions is good once the airway is secured. Epiglottitis is short-lived and, should tracheostomy be required in subglottic stenosis, as the child grows it is eventually always possible to remove the tracheostomy.

Mechanical ventilation in paediatrics

There are many reasons to institute artificial ventilation, and there are no rigid guidelines in paediatrics as in adult medicine. The indications vary widely with the age of the patient. In neonates, respiratory failure caused by congenital conditions affecting the lungs is easily the most common cause for artificial ventilation, while in older children primary respiratory problems are fewer.

Intubation

In prepubertal children the cricoid region of the trachea is the narrowest part of the airway and is at risk of damage by endotracheal intubation. Pressure on the mucosa will result in ischaemia and possible postextubation swelling and stridor or even permanent subglottic stenosis, which may be severe enough to require tracheostomy. Uncuffed endotracheal tubes are therefore used and should be sized correctly to allow a small leak of gas during inspiration, whilst allowing adequate inspiratory pressures to be obtained. The tip of the tube should be sited in the mid-trachea to avoid bronchial intubation or accidental extubation. As a small neonate may have a trachea shorter than 4 cm, correct judgement of length is essential, and should be confirmed by auscultation and X-ray for long-term ventilation.

Preformed tubes (e.g. RAE) do not allow for length adjustment, and suction catheters are difficult to pass. Shouldered tubes (e.g. Cole) may cause damage if they slip in too far and in any case have unfavourable gas-flow characteristics. They are favoured by some paediatricians for emergency resuscitation of the newborn but should be replaced for ventilation.

Straight tubes have the advantages of being able to be cut to length, allow the passage of suction catheters, and enable nasotracheal intubation, which is preferred for long-term use as it provides more secure fixation.

Ventilators

A paediatric ventilator should have the following features:

1. A good humidifier, able to deliver gases to the patient's lungs at over 36°C and nearly fully saturated.

2. Low volume and compliance of the circuit.
3. Either continuous gas flow or rapid response time for spontaneous breathing.
4. A wide range of respiratory rates and volumes.
5. Variable I:E ratio.
6. Display of pressure wave, taken from a point in the circuit near the patient.
7. A circuit which is light and easy to handle.
8. Variable flow rate.

There is no single ventilator which is ideal for all sizes of patient. Other factors such as reliability, ease of use, simplicity and personal preference also apply.

Types of ventilators

Positive pressure ventilators are almost universal. Negative pressure ventilators (e.g. 'iron lungs'), although more physiological in that air is drawn into the lungs by negative pressure as in normal breathing, are cumbersome, need a seal round the neck, and restrict nursing access.

Pressure-preset

The ventilator delivers gas to a preset pressure; the volume delivered to the patient will vary according to the characteristics of the circuit and the lung.

Neonates are usually ventilated by pressure-preset ventilators. The pressure in the patient's lungs has an almost square-wave pattern, i.e. it rises rapidly at the beginning of inspiration and then levels off. The flow of gas into the lungs is rapid at first and then tails away as the lungs fill. If there is a leak, the flow of gas in the circuit will be greater as the ventilator attempts to reach its preset pressure. Thus there is some compensation for the unknown leak around the uncuffed endotracheal tube. However, the actual alveolar ventilation is not known. The control of ventilation is initially by clinical judgement followed by the patient's response, both clinically and in terms of blood gases. Pressure-preset ventilation enables an upper limit to ventilatory pressure to be set, thus minimising barotrauma and reducing the chances of BPD developing. Peak airway pressures much over 25 cm H_2O cause pulmonary barotrauma.

Volume-preset

A fixed volume of gas is delivered; the pressure in the circuit and the patient's lungs varies, rising as the compliance falls.

Volume-preset ventilators are used to ventilate older children. Unlike infants and neonates, this group of patients does not have specialised ventilators, but ventilation with many adult ventilators is satisfactory. Some ventilators in this group have an adjustable flow pattern, but generally the flow is more constant and the increase in alveolar pressure and tidal volume more gradual than pressure-preset ventilators. Volume-preset ventilators do not compensate for variable leaks in the circuit. In small children the tidal volume is small compared to the circuit volume, and small tidal volumes may be difficult to set and to maintain constant when the lungs are abnormal. Some adult ventilators which normally function as volume preset have a pressure-preset mode to cope with this problem.

Most paediatric ventilators are time cycled, meaning that cycling from inspiration to expiration takes place after a certain fixed time. Other ventilators may be volume or pressure cycled. If there is a big leak around the endotracheal tube, volume-cycled ventilators may cycle without having achieved any alveolar ventilation, whilst pressure-cycled ventilators may not reach their cycling pressure and fail to cycle at all.

It is clear, therefore, that, at least for neonates and small infants, the best type of ventilator is time cycled and pressure preset. A ventilator should also have facilities for variable PEEP, and for IMV and CPAP.

Continuous positive airways pressure (CPAP)

This is used as the final weaning stage for infants and neonates coming off ventilation. It is also used for respiratory support for some patients who do not require full ventilation, such as mild cases of RDS, where early application of CPAP reduces the chance of ventilation being subsequently required. CPAP also reduces the number of apnoeas in premature infants, by improving oxygenation and stimulating stretch receptors.

CPAP may be delivered by tight-fitting mask or a headbox with neck seal. However, the most satisfactory methods are endotracheal tube or nasal prong. Except in the case of infants already intubated, a nasal prong inserted into one nostril is probably the easiest, although it occasionally causes gastric distension. (Nasal prongs work because neonates are obligate nasal breathers and cannot release the pressure through the mouth.)

CPAP is either applied from an appropriate ventilator or from a CPAP circuit. Whichever is used there should be a valve set to prevent excessive pressures. The flow of gas in the circuit should be sufficiently high to maintain a positive pressure at all stages of the respiratory cycle.

An initial pressure of 5 or $6\,cmH_2O$ is usually appropriate. CPAP pressures over $10\,cmH_2O$ are generally inadvisable as there is increased risk of pneumothorax and the cardiac output may fall.

Principles of ventilation

In the case of normally compliant lungs, a pressure-preset ventilator may typically be set at a peak pressure of about 14 or $15\,cmH_2O$, with a rate of 25 cycles per minute for an infant, 30 for a neonate and 20 for an older child. Poorly-compliant lungs will probably have been detected beforehand during initial hand ventilation, and in this case higher peak pressures should be set. Initial I:E ratios are normally between 1:1 and 1:1.5 with PEEP at $3-4\,cmH_2O$. The effectiveness of ventilation will be judged clinically at first, followed by blood gas analysis. The aim is to achieve optimal blood gases with the lowest FIO_2 and peak pressures.

In cases of severe RDS 'reversed I:E ratios' of 2:1 or 3:1 may be more effective than high pressures or high FIO_2 in improving blood gases. In older children on volume-preset ventilators, an initial tidal volume of $10\,ml/kg$ is usually more than enough, and will often need reducing in the light of blood gases. The initial FIO_2 can be the same as that prior to ventilation.

Babies frequently need sedation whilst ventilated, although adequate ventilation with some hypocarbia reduces the need, particularly in older children. Paralysis reduces the morbidity of high pressures from fighting the ventilator in patients with severe RDS. Paralysis is also used in ventilating head-injured patients. It is contraindicated to give muscle relaxants to conscious patients without also giving adequate sedation.

The physical surroundings of an intensive care unit may be frightening to older children, adding to the need for sedation. Parental visits and regular nursing by the same nurse may be helpful. Diurnal rhythms in neonates are disturbed by continuously-lit ITUs, after which it may take several months to regain normal circadian rhythms.

Ventilator-care of infants

Endotracheal tubes

A sign of a poor paediatric ITU is a high incidence of blocked or displaced endotracheal tubes. Nasotracheal tubes are easier to fix securely and are more acceptable to older children. Tube length should be checked radiologically. To avoid nasal damage from the connector, the end of the tube should protrude slightly, but not too far, to avoid kinking. Suctioning of endotracheal tubes should be 'clean', and the suction catheter passed as far as it will go, beyond the end of the endotracheal tube, withdrawn slightly, and suction applied. The suction catheter should not be so big as to block the endotracheal tube, otherwise atelectasis may ensue. A brief period of raised F_{IO_2} beforehand will reduce hypoxia during the procedure. It is not necessary to instil saline down endotracheal tubes prior to suctioning unless humidification is inadequate.

Humidification

This is essential, particularly for small infants and neonates. Gases should be supplied to the lungs at over 36°C and fully saturated. 'Rain out' or condensation in the tubing may be a problem, particularly if it tends to run into the patient or the ventilator. It can be reduced by newer humidifiers with heating elements in the tubing, or its effects reduced with water traps at the lowest point in the tubing.

Physiotherapy

Physiotherapy is generally assumed to be a good thing but there is sparse evidence that routine physiotherapy is of any use in preventing atelectasis. Ventilated infants should be turned regularly, every hour or two, the frequency depending on the severity of the illness. If collapse has occurred then physiotherapy should be applied regularly and frequently for the chest. Its duration should not be prolonged to the point where P_{aO_2} falls. Bronchoscopy has little place in treatment of collapse, or in dealing with secretions. It is difficult to perform in infants and neonates without causing marked hypoxia. Even the smallest fibreoptic bronchoscopes almost completely block the lumen of a neonate's endotracheal tube.

Monitoring

This is more necessary in paediatrics than in adults because of the rapidity of deterioration which may occur. Apart from the routine monitoring of ECG, BP and temperature, the following should be monitored:

- low-pressure alarms for disconnection
- airway pressure (visual display of waveform is best)
- inspired oxygen
- temperature of inspired gas.

Infection

An endotracheal tube increases the chance of infection, and another indicator of a good ITU is lack of cross-infection between patients. A low threshold for treatment of clinically-suspected infection should be maintained. However, interpreting the cultures of endotracheal aspirates is difficult as they often do not represent genuine infection.

Other aspects of care

Nutrition, fluid balance and temperature maintenance, for example, are essential for success.

Extracorporeal membrane oxygenation (ECMO)

This is technically feasible but expensive in money, time and skills. A catheter in either an internal jugular or femoral vein takes blood through an oxygenator and heat exchanger and the blood is then returned to the systemic circulation. It may have a role in the short-term treatment of cases such as diaphragmatic hernias with transitional circulations.

Bibliography

Section I. Cardiac medicine

Infective endocarditis

British Society for Antimicrobial Therapy (1982). Recommendations of a Working Party. *Lancet*, **ii**, 1323–1326

Krayenbuhl, H. and Rickards, A. (Eds) (1984). New aspects of bacterial endocarditis. *European Heart Journal*, **5** (Suppl. C), 1–146

Masur, H. and Johnson, W. (1980). Prosthetic valve endocarditis. *Journal of Thoracic and Cardiovascular Surgery*, **80**, 31

Nursing care

McCulloch, J., Townsend, A. and Williams, D. O. (1985). *Focus on Coronary Care: Modern Trends in Coronary Artery Disease*. pp. 189–190

Meltzer, L. E., Pinneo, R. and Kitchel, J. R. (1983). Balloon dilatation of coronary arteries: development of intensive coronary care. In *Intensive Coronary Care: A Manual for Nurses*, 4th edition, pp. 28–29

Advanced cardiovascular systems inc. (1985) – A patient's guide

Section II. Cardiac surgery

Myocardial protection during open heart surgery

Brown, A. H. (1982). The avoidance of reperfusion injury. In: *A Textbook of Clinical Cardioplegia*. Futura, New York

Valve surgery

Carpentier, A. (1983). Cardiac valve surgery: The French correction. *Journal of Thoracic and Cardiovascular Surgery*, **86**, 323

Cardiac transplantation

Copeland, D. and Stinson, E. (1980). Human transplantation. *Current Problems in Cardiology*, **3**, 4

Pennock, J., Oyer, P., Reitz, B. *et al.* (1982). Cardiac transplantation in perspective for the future: survival, complications, rehabilitation and cost. *Journal of Thoracic and Cardiovascular Surgery*, **83**, 168

Aortic aneurysms, dissection and peripheral vascular matters

Crawford, E. S. (Ed.) (1980). Progress in treatment of aortic aneurysms. *World Journal of Surgery,* **4**, 501

Crisler, C. and Bahnson, H.T. (1972). Aneurysms of the aorta. *Current Problems in Surgery,* **December**, 1–64

Hirst, A. E. Jr., Johns, V. J. Jr. and Kime, S. W. Jr. (1958) Dissecting aneurysm of the aorta: a review of 505 cases. *Medicine,* **37**, 217

Vecht, R. J. (1982). Dissection of the aorta. *British Journal of Hospital Medicine,* 656–660

Peri-operative infection in cardiac surgery

Abraham, E., Bland, R. D., Codo, J. C. *et al.* (1983). Sequential cardiorespiratory patterns associated with outcome in septic shock. *Chest,* **85**, 75

Carchmer, A. W. (1987). Prosthetic valve endocarditis. In *Current Therapy in Cardiovascular Disease,* Fortuin, N. (Ed.), Decker, Toronto, 155–158

Sheagren, J. W. (1988). Shock syndromes related to sepsis. In: *Cecil Textbook of Medicine.* (Eds J. B. Wynguarden and L. H. Smith), W. B. Saunders, Philadelphia

Sibbald, W. J. (1985). Myocardial function in the critically ill: factors influencing left and right ventricular performance in patients with sepsis or trauma. *Surgical Clinics of North America,* **65**, 867–889

Teply, J. F., Grunkemeice, F. L., Sutherland, H. D. *et al.* (1981). The ultimate prognosis after valve replacement: an assessment at 20 years. *Annals of Thoracic Surgery,* **32**, 111

Vert, T. S. A., Dismuker, W. E., Cobbs, G. C., Blackstone, E. H., Kirklin, J. W. and Berglochl, L. A. L. (1984). Prosthetic valve endocarditis. *Circulation,* **69**, 223

Section III. Paediatric cardiac disease

Paediatric postoperative care (general)

Insley, J. (1986). *A Pediatric Vade-Medicum,* Lloyd Luke, pp. 60–67

Roberton, N. R. C. (1986). *A Manual of Neonatal Intensive Care,* Edward Arnold, London, pp. 27–33

Index

305